INTERMITTENT FASTING FOR BEGINNERS

+

INTERMITTENT FASTING FOR WOMEN OVER 60

2 BOOKS IN 1

A Perfect Guide to Learn Why It Is Never Too Late to Start Fasting, with Delicious Recipes and Beginner-Proof Meal Plans to Slow Down Aging and Make the Fasting Easy

By

MELINDA FRANCIS

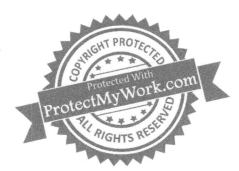

Table of Contents

INTERMITTENT FASTING FOR BEGINNERS

Chapter 1: What is Intermittent Fasting?

Intermittent fasting (IF) is an eating plan that alternates between fasting and normal mealtimes. According to studies, IF can aid in weight management and may even be able to reverse some diseases.

While many diets concentrate on what to eat, intermittent fasting only considers when to eat. In other words, you only eat within a specific time. Your body can burn fat if you fast for a set period each day or consume only one meal a couple of days a week. According to many researchers, our bodies have evolved to survive for several hours without eating, possibly several days or more. Before learning how to cultivate crops, early humans were hunters and gatherers who could live for extended periods without food.

It was simpler to maintain a healthy weight even 50 years ago. Christie Williams, M.S., R.D.N., a nutritionist at Johns Hopkins, explains: "There were no computers, and TV shows turned off at 11 p.m. In general, more people worked and played outside and got more exercise. TV, the internet, and other forms of entertainment are now accessible around-the-clock. We stay up late to play games, watch our favorite programs, and talk online. We spend most of the day and night lounging about and munching. An increased risk of obesity, heart disease, type 2 diabetes, and other ailments can result from eating more calories and being less active. According to scientific research, intermittent fasting might counter these tendencies.

There are various approaches to intermittent fasting, but they all start with deciding on regular eating and fasting windows time. According to Mattson, the body runs out of sugar after many hours without eating and begins to burn fat. He refers to this as metabolic switching.

"Intermittent fasting contrasts with the typical American eating habit, which involves eating throughout the day", claims Mattson. "If a person is eating three meals a day plus snacks and isn't exercising, they are burning off their fat storage instead of burning those calories every time they eat". Intermittent fasting extends when your body has burnt through the calories from your most recent meal and starts burning fat.

1.1 Intermittent Fasting Plans

It's essential to see your doctor before beginning an intermittent fasting plan. Once you get his approval, the actual practice is easy.

You can choose a strategy limiting daily meals to one six- to eight-hour window each day.

Consider trying the 16/8 fast, which involves eating for eight hours and fasting for sixteen. Williams advocates the daily routine, claiming that most individuals find it simple to maintain this pattern over time.

Another is the "5:2 approach", which calls for eating consistently five days a week and you restrict yourself to one 500–600 calorie meal on the other two days. For instance, if you decided to eat regularly every day of the week except for Mondays and Thursdays, which would be your one-meal days. Longer periods without food, such as 24, 36, 48, and 72 hours—are not always beneficial for you and may even be harmful.

If you go too long without eating, your body may begin accumulating extra fat as a defense against starvation. According to Mattson's studies, it might take the body two to four weeks to adjust to intermittent fasting. As you adjust to the new pattern, you can feel hungry or irritable. But he notes that once the adjustment period is through, research participants often continue with the strategy because they start to feel better.

What can I eat while intermittent fasting?

Water and zero-calorie drinks like black coffee and tea are OK while you aren't eating. Additionally, "eating properly" during your eating periods fill your mealtimes with high-calorie junk food, super-sized fried foods, and desserts.

Williams likes that intermittent fasting permits a variety of meals to be consumed and savored. She states that dining with friends and enjoying meals together increases enjoyment and promotes excellent health.

Williams agrees with most nutrition experts that whether you practice intermittent fasting or not, you can never go wrong when you choose complex, unprocessed carbs like healthy fats, lean protein, whole grains, and leafy greens.

Is intermittent fasting safe?

Some people experiment with intermittent fasting to lose weight, while others use the technique to treat long-term ailments, including high cholesterol, arthritis, or irritable bowel syndrome. But intermittent fasting isn't for everyone.

Some people should refrain from trying intermittent fasting:

- Children and teens under age 18.
- Women who are nursing or pregnant.
- Those who take insulin and have type 1 diabetes. There have been no tests in individuals with type I diabetes, despite an increasing number of clinical trials confirming the safety of intermittent fasting in those with type 2 diabetes. According to Mattson, there is a concern that an intermittent fasting eating pattern might lead to unsafe levels of hypoglycemia during the fasting phase because people with type I diabetes require insulin.
- Those with a history of eating disorders.

However, according to Williams, those who are not in these groups and can safely practice intermittent fasting can keep up the routine indefinitely. It can be a beneficial lifestyle change, she explains. Remember that different people may respond differently to intermittent fasting. Consult your doctor if you experience unusual anxiety, headaches, nausea, or other symptoms after beginning intermittent fasting.

1.2 How Different Is Intermittent Fasting From Other Diets

People who follow the plan intentionally alternate these "fasting" intervals with "feasting" moments during which they may eat everything they want.

One of the most enticing aspects of an IF eating plan is that no foods are forbidden, in contrast to most traditional diets that list certain foods to eat and avoid. You can often eat anything you want during the feasting phase. Caloric restriction (and its advantages) may be achieved without the difficulty of having to give up your favorite meals.

Calories

Following a time-restricted intermittent fasting strategy may allow you to consume enough calories to fulfill nutritional USDA recommendations. IF plans with time restrictions allow you normally eat at certain times of the day while fasting at other times. These plans often give you a 6–8-hour window to get the required calories. However, you won't be able to satisfy your caloric demands on specific days of the week with other forms of intermittent fasting.

For instance, diets like alternate-day fasting or the 5:2 plan severely restrict food intake on fasting days, so much so that you can only get a small portion of the calories you need for the day.

The 16/8 method, eat/stop/eat, alternate-day fasting, and Ramadan is more instances of intermittent fasting. The 16/8 method calls for a 14–16 hour fast daily with an 8–10 hour opportunity for eating.

Another approach is called "eat/stop/eat," in which you fast for 24 hours twice a week on different days. You are engaging in alternate-day fasting when you eat regularly one day and then very little to no calories the following. Muslims around the world observe fasting during the holy month of Ramadan. They observe fast from sunrise to sunset. The greatest research has been done on this fasting method.

These fasting plans may assist those who regularly consume too many calories in decreasing their weekly calorie consumption. On days when you fast, you consume extremely few calories. According to 2011 research, both methods of calorie restriction —intermittent fasting and continuous caloric restriction—are equally beneficial for helping obese and menopausal women lose weight. Age, gender, height, and degree of exercise are considered when the USDA recommends calorie intake. You can use a calorie calculator if you're unclear about how many calories you need to consume daily.

Food Groups

No food categories are forbidden or advised when following an intermittent fasting plan. However, it will be exceedingly challenging, if not impossible, to ingest the necessary amounts of several food categories on fasting days (but that's not the objective). It is extremely unlikely that you would be able to fulfill your recommended daily intake of calories or certain food categories when on an intermittent fasting eating plan. For instance, according to the 5:2 diet, a healthy woman should take 500 calories daily on fasting days. According to the USDA, a healthy woman should take 130 grams of carbohydrates daily. She only consumes more than 500 calories by following the USDA's suggested carb consumption. She would therefore be unable to eat any protein or healthy fat.

Additionally, some intermittent diet regimens recommend a total fast (almost no calories) during fasting days. Following such strategies would prevent a person from meeting any USDA-recommended consumption guidelines.

Similar Diets

There aren't many popular eating plans or diets that call for extended periods of total fasting. However, several well-liked diets incorporate periods of dietary restriction.

3-Day Diet

A group of diets collectively known as the "3-Day Diet" call for you to drastically restrict your calorie consumption for three days. For instance, those who adhere to the 3-Day Military Diet only eat a few things per meal that are minimal in calories.

Ease and Convenience: Most 3-day diets require you to adhere to a predetermined food plan during the program. This often involves going to the store and buying and measuring foods like hot dogs, saltines, grapefruit, or vanilla ice cream. This might not be convenient for some consumers.

Nutrition: Generally, most 3-day diets don't give your body the calories or nutrition required. Typically, people keep their caloric intake at 1,000 calories or fewer. Furthermore, maintaining these diets by consuming the necessary amounts of fruits, vegetables, and other healthy meals would be impossible. It is challenging to get your recommended daily allowance of vitamins and minerals from food alone while ingesting less than 1,200 calories daily. To follow this diet, taking supplements and getting help from a health expert, such as a registered dietitian nutritionist, will be necessary.

Health Benefits: Three-day programs are unlikely to offer any long-term health advantages. Any clinical studies do not support the efficacy of this diet.

Weight Reduction: A 3-day diet may result in temporary weight loss, but it is not likely to be sustained. Three days of a modified diet isn't likely to be enough to cause fat reduction. Instead, after resuming their usual eating habits, consumers may gain weight in fat while losing water and protein.

Body Reset Diet

Harley Pasternak, a famous fitness trainer, created the Body Reset Diet. You must go through a preliminary phase of the 15-day diet, during which food is strictly regulated. You avoid solid meals for the first five days and consume liquid smoothies. This portion of the diet has the sensation of a fast.

Ease and Convenience: Because the program only lasts 15 days, you must adhere to the instructions exactly if you want to see results. You frequently substitute liquid smoothies for whole-food meals. You also add some healthy solid foods throughout weeks two and three. Avoiding whole foods at mealtime in favor of smoothies may be difficult for some people. Also, exercise recommendations are provided. Although the recommendations are realistic, some people may find it challenging to alter their diet and increase their regular exercise simultaneously.

Nutrition: While following the Body Reset Diet, you will consume fewer calories than is recommended. You probably won't eat more than 1,200 calories daily throughout phase one. To help you feel satisfied, you will eat a balanced combination of protein, healthy fats, and carbohydrates. Recommended foods provide fiber and other healthy nutrients.

Health Benefits: This diet only lasts for 15 days. You are unlikely to experience any long-lasting health advantages during that little time. However, the program encourages an active lifestyle and offers recommendations for leaving the program. Your health may improve if you adhere to the advice and cut less on processed foods, red meat, and other unhealthy foods. However, there haven't been any clinical studies done.

Weight Loss: If you are inactive and eating a high-calorie diet before beginning, you will likely lose weight. Again, following the plan for only 15 days is unlikely to yield results you can maintain.

Fast Diet

Michael Mosley, a UK journalist with medical qualifications, created The Fast Diet, a variation of intermittent fasting. The eating plan uses a 5:2 eating approach, where you consume a "typical" diet five days per week and reduce your calorie intake on two days.

Ease and Convenience: This diet may be difficult for certain people to follow because the fasting days aren't followed by "feasting" days. You are encouraged to abide by calorie-restriction rules and take only enough calories to satisfy your energy demands on the days you are not fasting.

While no prohibited foods and a few little indulgences are permitted, many consumers who like intermittent fasting do so because they don't have to keep track of their calories and can eat anything they want on their non-fasting days.

Nutrition: This diet plan suggests eating healthy meals. On this diet, fasting days call for around 25% of your recommended daily calorie intake. That equates to around 500 calories for women and 600 calories for men. It would be impossible to consume the necessary amounts of key nutrients while remaining within that range.

Health Benefits: According to several studies that have looked at intermittent fasting, these regimens may lengthen life, improve heart health, and aid diabetics in controlling blood sugar. However, more extensive research is required to verify these advantages.

Weight Loss: Most research looking at intermittent fasting has revealed that weight loss is probably to happen. Studies have also revealed that the outcomes are not always superior to daily calorie restriction. Long-term research is also required to determine whether weight loss is sustained.

Master Cleanse Lemonade Diet

This rigorous diet promises weight loss of 10 pounds in just 20 days.

Ease and Convenience: While the program is simple, it is neither convenient nor simple. Those who adhere to the plan consume lemon-flavored beverages and saltwater throughout the day for ten days. They consume laxative-acting tea in the evening. Eliminating solid food is difficult for most people.

Nutrition: You cannot consume the required calories or nutrients while on this program due to the severe calorie restriction. You will probably consume much fewer daily calories when following the Master Cleanse Lemonade Diet, about 650 instead of the suggested 1,200.

Benefits to Health: It is unlikely that a short-term, extremely restricted program like this will positively affect health. The diet may cause health issues for you. Calorie restriction may cause fatigue, headaches, and dizziness. Furthermore, extreme hunger may lead to binge eating.

Weight Reduction: Any diet that forbids eating whole foods and caps daily calorie intake at 650 is likely to result in weight loss. But if you start eating normally again, weight reduction will probably not last. In addition to causing electrolyte imbalances and hair loss, these limitations also raise the risk of gallstones. Additionally, if you overeat after starting the program, you risk gaining back the lost weight.

1.3 Pros And Cons Of Intermittent Fasting

If you decide to try intermittent fasting, regardless of the method, it's crucial to concentrate on consuming nourishing meals like leafy greens and organic fruits and vegetables. It's important to remember that consuming processed food at meal times will prevent you from reaping the rewards of intermittent fasting. Like every diet, it has its benefits and drawbacks. Let's talk about the benefits and drawbacks of intermittent fasting.

Pros of Intermittent Fasting

Numerous studies show the wide variety of health advantages of intermittent fasting, including:

It Can Aid Weight Loss. As previously mentioned, fasting promotes ketogenesis, which enables your body to use stored fat as fuel rather than glucose. Your Human Growth Hormone (HGH), which is associated with fat reduction and muscle building, is increased by intermittent fasting.

In one research using alternate fasting days, patients shed an average of 8% of body fat in just eight weeks!

Insulin Resistance is reduced. According to research, prediabetics may benefit from intermittent fasting by having lower insulin levels and even better insulin sensitivity. According to one study, fasting considerably lowers blood sugar levels and increases weight reduction in type 2 diabetes patients.

It Can Reduce Inflammation. Chronic inflammation is at the root of almost every modern illness, including heart disease, diabetes, obesity, Alzheimer's, autoimmune disease, and cancer. There is good news, though! According to studies, fasting reduces levels of inflammatory cytokines and systemic inflammation. Additionally, it lessens oxidative stress, aiding your body in fending off dangerous free radicals.

It may reduce the risk of developing heart disease. According to studies, intermittent fasting can reduce the number of risk factors for heart disease. For instance, in one study, intermittent fasting reduced body fat, body weight, LDL cholesterol, triglycerides, and blood pressure. Adiponectin, a hormone with potent cardioprotective effects, is also produced in higher amounts during fasts.

It Promotes Brain Health. Fasting does not only benefit your heart; it helps your brain too! According to studies, intermittent fasting raises BDNF levels and may even promote the development of new neurons!
Low BDNF is associated with depression as well as cognitive impairment and decline. Fasting's anti-inflammatory effects might prevent Alzheimer's and other neurodegenerative diseases, but more study is required in this area.

It is Anti-Aging. Alterations in gene expression brought on by intermittent fasting promote lifespan and lower the risk of chronic disease. How? Fasting induces autophagy, your body's internal housekeeping system.

Your body eliminates old or damaged cells during autophagy and recycles the parts for cellular repair.

It Encourages Longevity. Increased autophagy may slow the aging process and lengthen life. Rats that fasted in one research on animals lived up to 83% longer!

Cons of Intermittent Fasting

Although there are many benefits to intermittent fasting, there are also some drawbacks. The drawbacks of intermittent fasting are listed below for you to consider before starting.

You Can Still Gain Weight. Intermittent fasting often results in a reduction in total calorie consumption. This is a crucial factor in the efficacy of intermittent fasting for weight loss. Many become frustrated with yo-yo dieting and switch to fasting to lose weight without worrying about calorie counts. If you overeat within your eating window, you can still risk putting on weight. Intermittent fasting does not permit you to eat piles of fast food. For the best outcomes, choose nutrient-dense meals like organic fruits and vegetables, grass-fed meat, wild seafood, and healthy fats for fuel.

There are Side Effects. Intermittent fasting may have negative impacts on certain people. This is especially the case when beginning intermittent fasting for the first time. As their bodies acclimate to calorie restriction, some people may develop what is known as a "fasting headache."
Other potential side effects include digestive issues (including nausea, constipation, diarrhea, & bloating), fatigue, dizziness, irritability, sleep disturbances, malnutrition, and dehydration.

It Can Influence Disordered Eating. Some people may develop harmful eating habits due to the restricted nature of intermittent fasting. For instance, intermittent fasting could cause binge eating when one is not fasting. This is especially true for persons who have a history of eating problems. If you struggle with disordered eating, fasting could be detrimental.

Intermittent Fasting Safety

Although intermittent fasting has many great health advantages, it's not for everyone. If you have any of the following conditions, discuss intermittent fasting with your doctor before starting.

- Diabetes or difficulty regulating blood glucose levels: Diabetic patients must often eat to check their blood sugar levels. If you have diabetes, intermittent fasting may result in dangerously low blood sugar levels. Intermittent fasting has been shown in studies to reduce blood pressure. Therefore, it may be risky for those with low blood pressure.

- Taking certain drugs: Exercise caution if you take blood pressure, thyroid, or diabetes medications. Fasting will affect their absorption. Many medications should also be taken regularly with meals. Consuming them while fasting may change absorption and heighten negative side effects.

- Underweight: If you are underweight, you will need enough consistent calories to keep your energy levels up.

- History of eating disorders: This has previously been said, but it is still important to note. If you have a history of disordered eating, kindly don't fast. Intermittent fasting may result in unhealthy eating habits like bingeing.

- Trying to conceive children: There is evidence that intermittent fasting may alter menstruation and affect fertility. Therefore, if you're trying to get pregnant, hold off on fasting.

- Pregnant or breastfeeding: It's difficult to get the nourishment you and your kid need during constrained eating times. It takes a lot of energy to feed or grow a human! Fasting might limit your nutrients and harm your baby's growth.

What to Consider Before Trying Intermittent Fasting

Intermittent fasting has benefits and drawbacks, but there are also dangers. As I've previously indicated, you should see your doctor before starting intermittent fasting. Several factors determine whether or not fasting is beneficial for you. Here are some things to consider before attempting intermittent fasting.

It's Not for Everyone. Fasting diets could worsen symptoms of hormonal imbalance, thyroid problems, and adrenal exhaustion. These effects are more severe in women because women's bodies are more sensitive to energy limitation than men's. In several studies, fasting resulted in irregular menstrual cycles. Energy restriction can also cause disturbances in sleep and hunger hormones. Fasting induces ketosis, which can stress your adrenal glands. Your adrenal glands and aids produce the stress hormone cortisol in preserving normal blood sugar levels.

If you have adrenal exhaustion, you will already struggle with blood sugar balance and cortisol production. See a functional medicine doctor if you have a medical issue that might be affected by fasting.

Start Slow. If you've never tried intermittent fasting, ease into it gradually. Start with longer eating intervals, like 12 hours. Then, pay attention to your body and gradually reduce your eating windows until you discover the one that works best for you. Spontaneous meal skipping can also be a simple initiation to fasting.

When you're not hungry or too busy to prepare a meal, simply skip it. A quick and easy approach to gradually acclimatize your body to longer fasting periods is to stop eating late-night snacks.

Provide Your Body with the Nutrients it Needs. It's essential to provide your body with the proper vitamins and nutrients for optimum health, especially during fasting. During your eating window, consume a lot of organic, nutrient-dense fruits and vegetables, wild seafood, and healthy fats. You will receive the nutrition you need from this to maintain your energy levels throughout the fasting time.

Adding a high-quality multivitamin can help fill up the gaps not covered by food alone. I recommend taking it with the first meal of the day to achieve the best absorption. Stress, persistent digestive problems, and soil depletion all influence our ability to meet our nutritional requirements. Getting all the vitamins, minerals, and nutrients needed throughout your fasting window might be difficult when you fast intermittently. That's why it's necessary to complement your diet with a potent, bioavailable multivitamin to satisfy your body's demands. Multivitamin provides a foundation for maximum health. It has the perfect ratio of chelated minerals, vitamin D, methylated B vitamins, and antioxidants to offer you all the nutrition your body needs.

Chapter 2: Types Of Intermittent Fasting

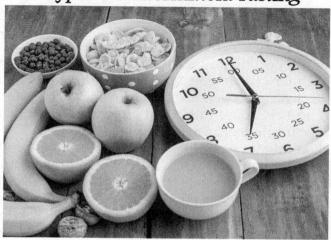

1. 5:2 Fasting
This is one of the most well-known IF methods. It was popularized by the best-selling book The FastDiet, which has all the information you want regarding this strategy. Eat normally for five days (don't watch calories) and then on the remaining two days, consume 600 or 500 calories per day for men and women, respectively.

Any days of your choosing may be used as fasting days. Short fasting periods are supposed to keep you compliant; if you are hungry on a fasting day, simply think of the next day when you can "feast" again. For certain people, a 5:2 approach could be more effective than calorie restriction for the full week. However, some authors warn against fasting on days when you could engage in vigorous endurance exercise.

If you're getting ready for a cycling or running race (or planning high-mileage weeks), examine whether this fasting form fits your training schedule. Or consult a sports nutritionist.

2. Time-Restricted Fasting

With this kind of IF, you select a daily eating window that, ideally, leaves a 14- to 16-hour fasting window. (Shemek advises women to fast for no more than 14 hours each day because of hormonal issues.) Fasting encourages autophagy, the body's natural "cellular housekeeping" process that eliminates waste and other obstructions to mitochondrial function, which starts when liver glycogen levels are low, according to Shemek. According to her, doing this could enhance fat cell metabolism and improve insulin performance.

This method allows you to select your eating window, for example, from 9 a.m. to 5 p.m. According to Kumar, it might be especially useful for someone with a family who already eats a late dinner. Then a large portion of the time spent fasting is sleep time. Depending on when you set your window, you theoretically don't have to "miss" any meals. But how consistently can you determine this? If your schedule is unpredictable, daily periods of fasting might not be for you.

3. Overnight Fasting

This strategy, the simplest of the lot, entails fasting every day for 12 hours. For instance, stop eating after supper at 7 p.m. and start again at 7 a.m. the following morning with breakfast. Autophagy does still occur at 12 hours mark, but the cellular advantages are less significant, according to Shemek. This is the bare minimum of hours she recommends fasting. The simplicity of this approach makes it beneficial.

Additionally, you don't have to miss meals; rather, all you are doing is forgoing a nightly snack (if you ate one, to begin with). However, this approach falls short of maximizing the benefits of fasting. If you are fasting to lose weight, a narrower fasting window gives you more time to eat, which may not assist you in reducing your calorie intake.

4. Eat Stop Eat

Author Brad Pilon invented this approach in his book Eat Stop Eat. His strategy is unique from others in that he emphasizes adaptability. In other words, he promotes that fasting is only a temporary respite from eating.

You commit to a resistance training regimen and execute one or two 24-hour fasts weekly. "When your fast is done, I want you to eat sensibly and act as if nothing ever happened. That's it. Nothing else," he says. To eat responsibly, one must return to a regular eating routine. This means avoiding binges after a fast but refraining from severe diets and eating less than necessary. Pilon says the optimal fat reduction regimen combines regular weight exercise with occasional fasting. You can eat more on five or six non-fasting days by allowing yourself to go on one or two 24-hour fasts during the week. Due to this, he says, finishing the week with a calorie deficit without feeling as though you must be on a strict diet is easier and more pleasurable.

5. Whole-Day Fasting
Here, you eat once a day. Shemek notes that some people opt to have dinner, then skip meals until the next day's dinner. In contrast to 5:2, where the fasting time is 36 hours, whole-day fasting involves fasting from dinner to dinner or lunch to lunch. The benefit of whole-day fasting for weight reduction is that it's extremely difficult, but not impossible, to consume all the daily calories at once. The drawback of this strategy is that it's challenging to get all the nutrients your body requires in one meal to function at its best. Not to mention, it might be difficult to maintain this strategy. You can be so hungry by supper that you make poor, calorie-dense food choices.
Consider this: When you're starving, broccoli isn't exactly what you want to eat. Shemek says that a large number of people also overindulge in coffee to stave off hunger, which can have a detrimental impact on your ability to sleep. You can also experience brain fog throughout the day if you aren't eating.

6. Alternate-Day Fasting
Krista Varady, Ph.D., a nutrition professor at the University of Illinois in Chicago, popularized this approach. A person may decide to fast every other day, consuming only 25% of their daily caloric needs (or around 500 calories) on the days they don't fast. This method of weight loss is popular.

Studies have shown that fasting on alternate days dramatically lowers body mass index, weight, fat mass, and total cholesterol in obese people. On fasting days, you might worry that you won't feel satisfied. Dr. Varady and colleagues' earlier studies showed that the hunger-related negative effects of alternate-day fasting started to subside by week two and began to improve by week four. The drawback of this strategy is that it might be difficult to stick to because research participants reported that they were never truly "full" during the eight-week experiment.

7. Choose-Your-Day Fasting

This kind of IF is more akin to choosing your adventure. According to Shemek, you might practice time-restricted fasting every other day or once or twice a week (for example, fast for 16 hours and eat for 8). This implies that Sunday may be a typical eating day, during which you finish eating at 8 p.m., and that you would start eating again on Monday at midday. In essence, it's similar to missing breakfast occasionally. Keep in mind that there is conflicting evidence about the impact of missing breakfast on weight loss. The possibility that missing breakfast impacts weight is not supported by compelling research. However, some studies have revealed that eating breakfast can only slightly affect weight reduction. But, several studies have linked skipping breakfast to a higher risk of mortality from cardiovascular disease. This approach may be more flexible and go with the flow, allowing you to make it work even if your schedule fluctuates weekly. But a looser approach could result in milder advantages.

2.1 How To Successfully Adapt Fasting Into Your Lifestyle

Fasting is a traditional food restriction practice that has gained popularity due to its numerous benefits for longevity, health, and weight loss. While it may seem hard to defy your body's urge to eat while fasting, we are returning to the hunter-gatherer lifestyle that required ancient people to endure days of protracted fasting. Fasting is still a demanding dietary change that is challenging to fit into the hectic modern lifestyle.

Different types of fasting

Caloric restriction has various positive health effects, including weight loss, defense against conditions like diabetes, cardiovascular disease, malignancies, and extended life span. It also has an impact on the processes of ketosis and autophagy. From casual meal skipping for those starting their fasting adventure to extreme 36-hour protracted fasts, there are several techniques to fit any lifestyle. Intermittent fasting (IF), which alternates between regular fasting and feasting, offers a happy medium and is especially simple to fit into busy lifestyles because it does not restrict your diet while eating.

There are many different types of intermittent fasting, including the 5:2 diet, where you restrict your caloric intake for two days a week and then eat as you please the rest of the time; the one meal a day fast (OMAD), also known as the "Warrior fast," where you only eat one large meal per day; and Time Restricted Eating (TRE), where you alternate fasting and feasting windows throughout the day.

TRE requires the least commitment because its fasting windows span from 12 hours with the simple 12:12 fast to 20 hours with the difficult 20:4 fast. One of the most popular TREs is the 16:8, which alternates 16 hours of fasting at night with 8 hours of eating during the day, following the body's natural circadian cycle.

Since it is practically impossible to eat while you are sleeping, most individuals complete some type of fast overnight! You can easily achieve the 16:8 by prolonging this natural fast by a few hours in the morning and evening.

Even if beginners generally avoid extremely protracted fasts, try out several fasting techniques until you discover the one that completely complements your way of life. In contrast to fad diets, fasting promotes long-term weight reduction by putting the body through food stress, which starts the metabolic state of ketosis (fat burning).

Setting realistic goals

Unlike fad diets, calorie restriction is a long-term weight loss approach that works over the long term by putting the body under nutritional stress and inducing the metabolic state of ketosis (fat burning). However, it is possible to go beyond and put the body under excessive stress, which can lead to weariness and mental exhaustion and negate the positive effects of fasting. For instance, attempting a 24-hour fast as a beginning to lose weight may result in adverse side effects. Instead, match your fast with your long-term weight loss objectives while remaining realistic.

Establish manageable intermittent fasting goals that are easier to reach than impossible prolonged fasting. For instance, a 12-hour fast once a week is a better compromise. Increase your fasting window or frequency after your first week of fasting, and keep doing so until you reach a comfortable level. If not, your body will be more equipped to withstand lengthy fasting by this point. By this time, you may already be satisfied with the weight reduction outcomes obtained by shorter fasts. It's easy to become fascinated with consuming food when your body adjusts to lengthy periods of fasting.

How to avoid eating during fasting

It is easy to become distracted with thoughts of food until your body adjusts to calorie restriction. Fortunately, there are various ways to prevent this, with preparation being the key. To guarantee that your social life does not interfere with your fast and vice versa, first write down your routine as well as any events that include eating. Then, arrange your fasting during these times.

When you schedule your fast around your social life, you can maintain your commitment to your fast and your friendships, as most human bonding occurs through food.

Making a shopping list and a cooking plan will help you have wholesome, satisfying meals available when it's time to break your fast. Eating healthily before your fast or during the feasting hours of an intermittent fast is another way to get ready to fast.

Before a fast, avoiding or limiting the consumption of sugars and refined carbs, which are found in sweets, soft drinks, and white bread, is beneficial. These meals have a detrimental influence on how the body metabolizes fat. Instead, choose the traditional Mediterranean diet, which provides the ideal ratio of fish protein, low glycemic carbs from vegetables, and healthy fats from olive oil to complement your selected fast.

This will also make you feel fuller for longer while consuming fewer calories.

Allow yourself the odd indulgence by including your favorite meals and snacks during your feasting hours if it helps you stay committed to your fast—always in moderation.

It's important to limit how much you eat when you can eat. When you overcompensate for periods of fasting by consuming large, high-calorie meals during periods of feasting, your body will use up energy to process the abrupt reintroduction of food, which can make you feel tired. You can maintain control over your eating by controlling portion sizes, and practicing intermittent fasting can even make you feel less hungry. It's important to stay active when fasting because boredom triggers increased consumption of unhealthy foods. For instance, upping your exercise regimen while on a calorie-restricted diet can increase your fast's health benefits while keeping your body and mind active and preventing food cravings.

While it is not advised to engage in vigorous activity while fasting, gentle cardiovascular exercises like yoga and walking, as well as strength-based workouts for no more than an hour each day, are ideal. You can avoid overeating while on a fast by adding a new workout routine or activity to your schedule. This will also help you reach holistic health. Finally, let people know your calorie restriction objectives so they can support you and keep you on track. This can be family or coworkers at work, Depending on the time of day your fast falls. This will make you more accountable for achieving your weight reduction objectives, and if you succeed, it could even convince others to adopt a fasting lifestyle!

Chapter 3: Foods To Eat And Limit On An Intermittent Fasting Diet

3.1 Foods to eat
The foods you should be sure to consume on an IF diet comes from the following food groups:

- Lean proteins
- Fruits
- Vegetables

Lean proteins
According to Maciel, fasting is important to eat lean protein because it makes you feel fuller for longer than other foods and helps you keep or gain muscle.
Examples of lean, healthy protein sources include:

- Plain Greek yogurt.
- Chicken breast.
- Fish and shellfish.
- Beans and legumes, like lentils.
- Tofu and tempeh.

Fruits
As with any diet plan, eating various nutrient-dense meals while intermittent fasting is important. Vitamins, minerals, phytonutrients (plant nutrients), and fiber are frequently abundant in fruits and vegetables.
These nutrients, vitamins, and minerals can support intestinal health, blood sugar regulation, and cholesterol reduction. Fruits and vegetables are low in calories, which is another benefit. According to the 2020-25 Dietary Guidelines for Americans, most adults should consume roughly 2 cups of fruit per day to maintain a 2,000-calorie diet.

When intermittent fasting, try to eat certain kinds of fruit, for example:

- Apricots.
- Apples.
- Blackberries.
- Blueberries.
- Cherries.
- Pears.
- Plums.
- Peaches.
- Melons.
- Oranges.

Vegetables

Vegetables can be an essential part of an IF regimen. According to research, a diet high in leafy greens may lower your chance of developing heart disease, cancer, Type 2 diabetes, cognitive decline, and other diseases. According to the government's 2020-25 Dietary Guidelines for Americans, most individuals should consume 2.5 cups of vegetables per day for a diet of 2,000 calories.

Affordable veggies that can work on an IF protocol include:

- Broccoli.
- Carrots.
- Cauliflower.
- Tomatoes.
- Green beans.

Leafy greens are also a great option because they are full of nutrients and fiber. Consider including these options in your diet:

- Arugula.
- Spinach.

- Kale.
- Cabbage.
- Chard.
- Collard greens.

3.2 Foods to Limit on an Intermittent Fasting Diet

Some meals aren't as good to eat as part of an intermittent fasting plan. Foods that are heavy in calories, saturated fat that is bad for your heart and salt should be avoided. After a fast, "they won't fill you up and can even make you hungry," claims Maciel. Furthermore, they offer very little to no nutrition.

Limit the following foods to maintain a healthy intermittent eating schedule:

- Snack chips.
- Pretzels and crackers.
- Meals that include a lot of added sugar. According to Maciel, processed sugar is nutritionally worthless and only provides sweet, empty calories, which is not what you want if you're occasionally fasting. They will make you feel hungry because sugar metabolizes so quickly.

The following are some examples of sugary foods you should avoid during intermittent fasting:

- Candies.
- Cakes.
- Cookies.
- Highly sweetened coffee and teas.
- Fruit drinks.
- Sugary cereals with little fiber and granola.

INTERMITTENT FASTING FOR WOMEN OVER 60

Introduction

Intermittent fasting has become popular in recent years due to its range of health benefits and not restricting your food choices. According to research, fasting can help you lose weight, enhance your mental health, and help avoid certain malignancies. It can also help prevent certain muscle, nerve, and joint diseases in women over 60.

Adults who practice intermittent fasting can experience weight loss and reduce the risk of acquiring age-related ailments. According to a new study by Baylor College of Medicine, intermittent fasting can help reduce blood pressure levels. According to the study's findings, fasting can reduce blood pressure by altering the gut flora.

Of course, Women over the age of 60 are concerned about losing weight and trying to improve their health. It is more difficult to lose weight after age 60 for various reasons, including decreased metabolic rate, achy joints, muscle mass, and even sleep troubles. Meanwhile, lowering weight – particularly hazardous belly fat – can significantly lower your chance of developing major health problems such as diabetes, heart disease, and cancer.

Of course, as you become older, your chances of having a variety of ailments grow. In certain situations, intermittent fasting for women over 60 can act as a genuine fountain of youth when it comes to weight loss and reducing the risk of acquiring age-related ailments such as heart disease and diabetes.

Chapter 1: Ways Your Body Changes As You Age

Long life is a blessing that some never get to experience. But for those who do, that blessing is accompanied by certain inescapable aging symptoms. Your body changes as you age, which is not always bad; it's simply different.

Understanding what to expect can help you welcome these changes and alert you to what you can do to speed up the process. While some of these changes may be gradual and subtle, others may appear to occur suddenly. No matter when they occur, it's critical to understand that they're normal.

Ways Your Body Changes As You Age
Change #1: Cardiovascular System

Your heart and blood arteries grow more inflexible as you age, and the heart fills with blood less quickly. The more inflexible the arteries are, the less room they have to expand as blood is pushed through them, which is why older persons are more likely to develop high blood pressure. A healthy older heart still functions normally, but it simply cannot pump as much blood or at the same rate as a younger heart. Because of this, older athletes often don't perform as well as younger ones. The death rate from heart-related disorders has decreased due to the numerous medical advancements accomplished during the past 20 years. As you age, your heart and arteries get more rigid; therefore, it's critical to take all reasonable steps to maintain the health of your cardiovascular system. A nutritious diet and physical activity, particularly aerobic exercise, are two excellent ways to accomplish this.

Change #2: Lungs

As you become older, your rib cage's muscles and diaphragm weaken. Additionally, the lungs lose some of their elasticity, reducing the amount of oxygen that is inhaled. This can make breathing challenging for smokers or anyone with a lung disease. Your lungs lose their ability to fend off illnesses as they deteriorate. These bacteria might linger and cause issues because they cannot spread germs without a good stiff cough.

The two best activities you can engage in to enhance lung health are:

- Avoid smoking
- Regularly engage in aerobic activity of some kind. Exercise will provide your lungs the greatest opportunity to continue supplying your body with oxygen allowing you to stay active because your lungs aren't what they once were.

Change #3: Immune System

As you age, your immune system becomes less effective, raising your risk of getting sick. Vaccines like those for the flu and pneumonia could not be as effective or durable as they once were. Because you have fewer immune cells as you age, your body recovers itself more slowly. You have a higher chance of getting cancer because as you become older, your body becomes less capable of identifying and repairing cell flaws. An autoimmune illness is one where your immune system unintentionally targets and kills healthy bodily tissue. It's essential to take good care of yourself to help you keep your immune system as strong as possible.

Get the vaccines your doctor advises, such as those for pneumonia, shingles, pneumococcal disease, and the flu. You can maintain a balanced diet, exercise, quit smoking, and consume less alcohol while building a robust immune system.

Change #4: Urinary Tract

The urinary tract system often continues to function normally, barring any diseases or illnesses that affect it. If you're over 60, you've undoubtedly realized that you have to get up at least once throughout the night to use the bathroom. This is typical for this age group because as you get older, your bladder's capacity declines. Additionally, when the bladder muscles deteriorate, it may become harder to empty your bladder and shut the urinary sphincter, which might lead to leakage.

These problems may lead to urinary incontinence. Some drugs can help with these issues, as well as pelvic floor (Kegel) exercises and bladder training.

Change #5: Bones and Joints

Your bones and joints start to age beyond the age of 60. You absorb less calcium from your diet as you become older. Without calcium, your bones deteriorate and become brittle and feeble. Your body's ability to metabolize calcium is aided by vitamin D, which declines with age. Osteopenia (moderate loss of bone density) or osteoporosis may arise from a drop in calcium and vitamin D levels (severe loss of bone density). When osteoporosis appears, your chance of fracture and break increases significantly. Osteoporosis may be avoided by maintaining a healthy weight and engaging in weight-bearing exercises to promote bone density. You might want to discuss calcium and vitamin D supplements with your doctor.

Physical Changes As You Age

After many years of usage, your joints' surrounding cartilage may thin out, making movement painful. This cartilage deteriorates with time, making mobility difficult and perhaps dangerous.

Osteoarthritis, a fairly common aging condition, may eventually develop from this. Unfortunately, wear and tear from years of usage causes joint discomfort, and surgery is now the only option to reverse it. Your doctor might occasionally recommend vitamins to aid with the discomfort. You might want to bring up this during your next appointment.

Change #6: Muscle Tone and Body Fat

Around 30, your body begins to develop fat and lose muscle tone. The loss of muscle mass can be pretty substantial by the time you reach 60.

According to MedilinePlus, only approximately 10 to 15% of muscle mass is lost as people age. The rest is a result of inactivity and a poor diet. The good news is that you can maintain or improve your muscle tone even after you become 60.

1.1 Ways Your Body Changes After You Turn 60

Strength training, often known as resistance training, is essential to maintaining and regaining muscular tone via regular exercise. Eating healthily goes hand in hand with regular exercise. Together, these two substances can reduce body fat and improve muscular tone. With aging, body fat tends to rise. In this period of life, it's simple to develop a sedentary lifestyle as a habit. It's simple to develop the daily habit of doing virtually nothing, especially nothing physical because you become tired more quickly than you used to. Your chance of having diseases like diabetes is elevated by increased body fat. You can maintain a healthy body fat percentage by exercising regularly and eating a balanced diet.

Change #7: Eyesight

You'll likely notice a difference in your vision by age 60. You could notice changes in your sense of color, a loss of close vision, and an increasing need for stronger lighting to read and discern details. These are generally caused by the lenses in your eyes stiffening and turning yellow.

Your eyes may experience various physical changes as you age:

- Your eyes' whites can start to turn yellow.
- The whites of your eyes may develop a few specks of color.
- A gray-white ring may appear around the surface of the eye.

Muscle loss may cause your lower lid to start drooping. If you lose fat around your eyes, it might make your eyes look sunken. You'll probably notice as you get older that your eyes are often dry. To solve this issue, lubricating eye drops can be used. These changes to your eyes and vision are consequences of aging. See an eye doctor if they are painful or if you detect a significant change.

Change #8: Hearing

Some hearing loss is not genuinely age-related; rather, it results from environmental exposure over time.

Age-related hearing impairments, though, exist, such as the inability to perceive high-pitched noises. With aging, one's ability to detect high-pitched noises significantly decreases. Presbycusis is the name given to this age-related hearing loss. The ability to grasp what others are saying is the biggest problem with presbycusis.

Consonants are difficult to hear because they are often uttered in a higher tone than vowels, caused by a mix of high-pitched voices, mainly those of women and children. Unfortunately, it ultimately gets harder to detect lower-pitched tones as well.

Aging Is Real. Hearing difficulties might also result from earwax buildup and background noise. You can improve your hearing by maintaining clean ears and wearing hearing aids.

Change #9: Teeth

As you reach 60, cavities become a major problem, mostly because of dry mouth. Dry mouth is not a problem exclusive to old age, but it is a side effect of many medications older people take for other illnesses. Gum disease is another problem that frequently arises at any stage of life, especially as you age. While it is painless, if addressed, it can result in several issues, including tooth loss. After 60, mouth cancer becomes a risk as well. Oral cancer typically has no discomfort in its early stages, and early identification can save lives. After age 60, your body will undergo physical changes.Your mouth, gums, and teeth can all benefit greatly from routine dental checkups. Early diagnosis saves money while also saving lives.

Change #10: Skin

Your skin changes as you get older. It gets drier, thinner, less elastic, and more wrinkled.

Many things in the skin start to decrease, such as elastin, collagen, the layer of fat under the skin, nerve endings, sweat glands, blood vessels, and pigment-producing cells. The lack of these things causes your skin to become easily bruised and torn, sag and bag, crack and peel, and get age spots and wrinkles.

A reduced sensitivity to discomfort also raises your risk of experiencing a heat stroke.

1.2 Body Changes After 50 and 60

You may be at risk for vitamin D insufficiency once you become 60 because your skin can no longer produce vitamin D from exposure to sunshine.

If you want to prevent this problem, discuss taking a supplement with your doctor. Even while it's best to take care of your skin when you're young, there are still things you can do to protect it in the future. You can start using moisturizers and sunscreen, undergo surgical procedures like laser treatments, and your doctor may prescribe prescription drugs like hydroquinone for aging spots.

Accepting Physical Changes After 60

Aging is a privilege. Many people have remarked that they would have taken better care of their bodies if they had known they would live thus long. That sentence undoubtedly has a lot of truth for several people.

While there is nothing you can do to change what you did or didn't do in the past, you can go forward and take the best possible care of yourself right now. Practically all aspects of your evolving physique may be improved with regular exercise and a healthy diet. So stay active, eat healthily, and enjoy the rest of your life.

1.3 Benefits Of Intermittent Fasting For Women Over 60

Not only does intermittent fasting support your waistline, but the risk of developing various chronic diseases may also be decreased.

Heart Health

One study of sixteen obese men and women found that intermittent fasting decreased blood pressure by 6 percent in just eight weeks.

The same research also found intermittent fasting decreased 25 percent of LDL cholesterol and 32 percent of triglycerides. However, the evidence for the correlation between intermittent fasting and improved LDL cholesterol levels and triglycerides is inconsistent. Until researchers can fully understand the effects of intermittent fasting on heart health, higher-quality studies with more rigorous methods are needed.

Diabetes

Intermittent fasting can also help to control and reduce the risk of developing diabetes effectively. Intermittent fasting tends to decrease some risk factors for diabetes, comparable to constant calorie restriction. This is achieved primarily by reducing insulin levels and reducing insulin resistance.

However, intermittent fasting might not be as effective for women as men in terms of blood sugar. A small study found that after 22 days of alternate-day fasting, blood sugar regulation worsened for women, although there was no adverse effect on men's blood sugar. Despite this side effect, insulin and insulin resistance reductions are still likely to decrease the risk of diabetes, particularly for people with pre-diabetes.

Weight Loss

When done correctly, intermittent fasting can be a quick and efficient way to lose weight, as daily short-term fasting can help you eat fewer calories and shed pounds. Several studies show intermittent fasting for short-term weight loss is as effective as conventional calorie-restricted diets.

A 2018 study of overweight adults' studies showed that intermittent fasting resulted in an average weight loss of 15 lbs (6.8 kg) over 3-12 months. Another review found intermittent fasting decreased body weight by 3-8 percent in overweight or obese adults over 3-24 weeks. The evaluation also showed that participants decreased their waist circumference by 3-7% over the same period.

Note: The long-term effects of intermittent fasting on weight loss for women remain to be seen.

Intermittent fasting tends to help in weight loss. However, the amount you lose will depend on how many calories you eat during non-fasting periods and how long you stick to the lifestyle.

Other Health Benefits
Various studies indicate that intermittent fasting may yield other health benefits.

- **Reduced inflammation:** Some study shows that intermittent fasting can decrease main inflammation markers. Chronic inflammation may contribute to weight gain and various health issues.

- **Improved psychological well-being:** One study found that depression and binge eating habits were reduced after eight weeks of intermittent fasting while enhancing body image in obese adults.

- **Increased longevity:** It has been shown that intermittent fasting increases lifespan by 33-83% in rats and mice. The effect on human survival has yet to be calculated.

- **Preserve muscle mass:** In contrast to constant calorie restriction, intermittent fasting tends to be more efficient at maintaining muscle mass. Even at rest, higher muscle mass lets you consume more calories.

Chapter 2: Exercising While Fasting

Working out while on an intermittent fasting (IF) plan could seem very difficult. If you've ever gone without food for a long time, you know that it can sometimes leave you feeling weak, tired and - of course - extremely hungry. But lots of people laud the advantages of fasted cardio. So, how can your IF plan and your workout plan be safely and effectively combined?

Here is a detailed guide on exercising on IF without sacrificing your long-term health objectives.

Can you exercise while observing an intermittent fast?

Yes, to answer briefly. The longer response is that it is dependent upon your mood. According to Vincent Pedre, M.D., a functional medicine doctor who frequently suggests IF to his patients, "It's vital to listen to your body." It all boils down to creating a strategy that works well for you, as with most things. The 16:8 plan and the 5:2 plan are two examples of the several IF variations.

To acquire the nutrients your body requires, you'll need to modify your fast based on your chosen workout type and the time of day you prefer to exercise. If you feel too weak to exercise from fasting, Pedre advises taking care of your nutrition first and working out afterward. This is especially true when it comes to exercising during fasting, which offers both advantages and possible disadvantages.

Benefits of working out while fasting

When you get out of bed and go to your 7 a.m. spin class, you probably haven't eaten anything since dinner the previous night. This type of cardio exercise may help you achieve your weight loss goals.

A 2016 research published in the Journal of Nutrition and Metabolism indicated that exercising when fasting can enhance fat oxidation1, which implies that your body is using its fat reserves as energy rather than the carbohydrates from your most recent meal.

Generally, it's better to gauge how you feel when choosing whether fasted workouts are your thing. Try out a few different daily workout schedules without hesitation to find one that you can easily maintain.

Things to look out for

If exercising on an empty stomach makes you feel great - more power to you! - continue with what works for you. But be aware that it may be time to change your routine if you start to feel weak or dizzy throughout your workout. Working out while fasting might help you lose more fat, but it can also cause you to lose more muscle, according to Jaime Schehr, N.D., R.D. If the body's glycogen stores (often known as its energy stores) are low, the reverse of what most people are aiming for might happen. If you want your muscles to get stronger and prevent damage, you must replenish your body with carbs and protein (especially soon after working out).

2.1 How to choose the best exercise for your IF plan

Not every workout is the same when scheduling an exercise with your intermittent fasting regimen. Some forms of exercise are more likely to deplete your muscles than others, so you might need to eat right away or consume more carbohydrates earlier in the day. Cardio and HIIT Fasted cardio may be a beneficial addition to your fitness routine when done properly. And depending on the kind of exercise you undertake, you might or might not need to eat right away.

According to Schehr, who speaks to mbg, "I usually advise my clients that if it was a high-intensity interval training cardio with perhaps some strength-based component to it, we want it closer to when they would break their fast".

Contrarily, if it's more of a steady-state cardio, it may not be as close to breaking the fast. If you plan to run slowly and steadily in the morning, you might be able to wait many hours before eating.

However, if doing that makes you feel weak and lightheaded, consider eating right after your workout. It's also vital to ease into any rigorous exercise when following this new diet.

"Easing into fasted cardio might take some time if people have a lot of hypoglycemia and don't feel well when fasting," adds Schehr". To enter these fasting states, your body has to be trained." She advises gradually increasing the intensity of your exercises as your body adjusts to doing out while fasting.

Exercise for muscle

Fueling your body with protein and complex carbs before working out or just after is crucial to gaining muscle mass. If someone wants to increase mass and strength, Schehr advises that they should work out either soon before they break their fast or throughout their eating window rather than towards the end because they won't recover.

By performing your strength training during your eating window, you can ensure that your muscles have enough fuel to function properly. According to Abby Cannon, J.D., R.D., CDN, the key is to do what makes you feel the best. "What are your workout goals? We sort of have to strike a balance" she claims. "If you discover that working out leaves you feeling completely exhausted, something is wrong.

If you want to achieve your weightlifting or HIIT workout goals, you could benefit from eating a small portion of food beforehand". In this situation, your plan will work best if you exercise in the afternoon or evening.

Yoga, barre, and low-intensity workouts

Low-intensity workouts, whether done fasted or within your eating window, might be gentler on your body when you're feeling low on energy or when you are first adjusting to intermittent fasting. According to Schehr, these can be fantastic alternatives if you're looking for a quick exercise to fit within the fasted window of your day". Those often do significantly better fasted [than strength training], "She clarifies.

When doing exercises like pilates, yoga, or barre within their fasting window, those who wish to practice intermittent fasting a few times per week perform considerably better than those who need to be able to replace their nutrients and protein during strength- or high-intensity-based workouts.

2.2 Your 7-Day Exercise Plan

Monday: morning cardio followed by a breakfast high in protein.

Tuesday: complex carbohydrates for lunch, weight training in the evening, and dinner.

Wednesday: a low-intensity workout such as yoga, Pilates, or barre

Thursday: morning cardio followed by a breakfast high in protein.

Friday: complex carbohydrates for lunch, followed by weight training in the evening and dinner

Saturday and Sunday: Yoga, Pilates, barre, or any low-intensity exercise

This program is based on your fasting requirements and can be modified to suit your needs.

Tips for working out while intermittent fasting

Ease into it. Try increasing your workouts gradually as your body gets used to this new eating regimen, as no ideal strategy will work for everyone. According to Cannon, if you are used to eating before exercising, an hour-long workout in the morning will be too much. However, if you complete a little exercise of only 15 or 20 minutes, you might get away with it during the transition.

Consider what time of day you like to exercise. If you only work out pre-8 a.m, you may need to change your eating schedule so you can eat right after a cardio session. If you enjoy working out in the late afternoon, it is the best time for weight training. You can work out at low intensity at any time of day.

Your eating window should be flexible. If you enjoy morning runs as much as your friend does, sticking to an eating window of 12 pm to 8 pm won't be as effective. You might need to change your eating schedule to a 9 am to 5 pm time-frame to fit in a post-workout protein shake.

Hydrate. You shouldn't skimp on the water just because you are going a long time without eating! "Making sure you stay hydrated when performing fasted exercise is essential for someone who practices intermittent fasting," according to Schehr. Drink at least 72 ounces of water daily if you sweat a lot.

Use electrolytes. Natural sports drinks or other low-calorie solutions like coconut water can ensure that your body is replenished with electrolytes without breaking your fast.

Vary your workouts. Your body will benefit from a combination of strength training and cardio to help you burn fat and develop muscle. You could also use this to aid with your IF schedule.

Cardio should be your main emphasis on days you can work out in the morning; on days you have to go to the gym in the evening, strength training should be your best friend. Skip your workout when you're exhausted, and try yoga or Pilates instead.

Listen to your body. The exercise plan that leaves you feeling energized and powerful rather than weary is ultimately the one that is ideal for you. Schehr states, "Whatever will make us feel better is our body's indicator of what's best for us." Do not push yourself to the point of fatigue to take that spin class four times a week.

What if I want to try the 5:2 or an alternate-day fast?
Schehr advises doing a modest, low-intensity workout (or no workout) when your fasting plan demands significant calorie restriction. "I wouldn't put anything likely to enhance caloric expenditure on a day when you are trying to cut calories," she advises. What justifies this? You don't want to expend more calories than you need to, further depleting your body. "You force yourself into a condition of depletion when you start adding exercise to a daily activity with just 500 calories," she notes. "This might make you more drained, tired, less likely to recover, and higher risk for injury." Therefore, a person following the 5:2 plan should alter their routine to ensure that their main workouts occur during the five days when they are eating and are less intense during the two days they are fasting. Once more, experiment a little to discover what works for you. And remember that intermittent fasting simply entails eating on a schedule rather than less often. According to Schehr, fasting does not entail not eating. It implies consuming your recommended daily calories and nutrition within a set window. She clarifies how the myth of "skipping meals" could harm the end goal of IF. Ensuring that the diet is optimized during that feeding window is what we want to achieve, she explains. "And then you'll receive the finest results".

Try out various exercise routines to see what you can maintain, and always believe your body is telling you what it can handle.

2.3 Yoga And Intermittent Fasting

Yoga practitioners are likely to pay special attention to their health and wellness, with weight control playing a significant role in this. As a result, it is not unusual to find many yoga practitioners interested in diets and weight loss. Although it's a common practice, many people ask if intermittent fasting is appropriate for practicing yoga.

When done properly, intermittent fasting for weight loss is acceptable for yoga practitioners. The two procedures are typically safe for most individuals, while special precautions may be needed for pregnant women with eating problems or certain sorts of injuries.

It will be helpful to evaluate the two disciplines in more detail to determine how to combine these two practices for optimal advantage and safety. In this chapter, we'll examine the objectives and results of yoga compared to those of intermittent fasting. We'll be able to clearly understand how the two work best together, where they might contradict, and how to work through those issues for your benefit.

Yoga

Yoga is a term used to describe a collection of disciplines or practices that have roots in India but have since developed into a kind of posture-based physical exercise, relaxation, and stress-relieving methods. In the West, many styles of yoga are frequently practiced, with some stressing the physical (hatha) and others focusing more on the mental and spiritual (mantra, laya). It is a holistic practice because it attempts to help the mind, body, and spirit. Asanas, or the positions we most commonly identify with yoga, are used in concert with meditation and regulated breathing (ujjayi or pranayama) to create a perfect yoga session.

There are a lot of well-known benefits of practicing yoga, such as:

1. Weight loss
2. Inflammation reduction
3. Stress relief

4. Anxiety relief
5. Alleviate depression
6. Improve heart health
7. Ease chronic painImprove breathing
8. Improve balance
9. Increase flexibility
10. Promote healthy eating habits
11. Improve quality of life
12. Increase cognitive function (mental abilities)

Weight Loss Effectiveness

Before looking at what else these two disciplines can do for us, we'll thoroughly examine this aspect, as weight reduction and weight control are the main reasons why most people are interested in intermittent fasting. Yoga can be used successfully as a natural and long-lasting workout program for weight loss and weight management. Variations of hatha yoga that strongly emphasize postures (asanas) and controlled breathing (pranayama) might aid in weight loss in various ways. his study thoroughly goes into yoga's physical, behavioral, and psychological impacts that contribute to weight reduction.

Weight Loss Through Physical Exertion

Some well-liked yoga types are Ashtanga, Bikram (hot), Iyengar, and Kundalini. These types use dynamic, flowing movements (vinyasa), rhythmic breathing, and postures to provide great aerobic exercise. Some of these programs allow you to burn as many calories as a rigorous cycling, running, or swimming session.

However, it must be acknowledged that the effectiveness of yoga as a weight-loss strategy depends partly on the practitioner's present physical state and level of expertise.

Even while they may undoubtedly benefit in other ways, an unfit beginner to yoga may not have the strength and expertise to fully reap the benefits of a good session regarding weight reduction.

Weight Loss Through Increased Mindfulness

Others believe that the principle of mindfulness that yoga instills in us is the most fundamental way yoga helps us on our weight loss journeys, even though some swear by the effectiveness of physically demanding yoga for weight reduction. Mindfulness is the conscious ability to observe what happens in our bodies objectively and non-reactively. We can notice and alter our relationship to food and eating thanks to the mind-body connection at the core of yoga practice. Yoga practitioners will find it easier to make the regular and habit adjustments that an intermittent fasting program would need. It is easier to resist destructive eating habits and desires when you are more aware of your body and its functions.

Ideal Yoga Practice Times While Intermittent Fasting

The best time to practice yoga while fasting intermittently is a topic of much debate. It is a valid concern because we don't want to risk unintentionally endangering our health while trying to better ourselves. To answer the question, doing yoga before or just after your fasting hours is advised. Your body will have plenty of energy reserves saved up in the hours before fasting to get you through your yoga practice, no matter how challenging. You could be on an empty stomach after your fasting hours, but you can eat something after your workout to replenish your energy. Many people believe that exercising or practicing yoga on an empty stomach has a larger impact on weight reduction since it forces the body to burn fat to meet its energy demands. This phenomenon is known as metabolic switching.

Stress Relief Effectiveness

Yoga is a well-known method for reducing stress and is preferred by people who desire an all-natural remedy without using drugs or other chemicals. While you might think that the calming and contemplative kinds of yoga, like yin yoga or Kriya yoga, are the ones to consider for stress relief, even the more physically demanding types of yoga, like Ashtanga and hot yoga, can be helpful. Most types of yoga use physical positions and breathing techniques to relieve stress, anxiety, and depression. Yoga's major mechanism of action in this respect is its capacity to lessen the levels of the stress hormone cortisol released into our bodies.

Yoga and Intermittent Fasting are compatible with reducing stress. If reducing stress is your top priority, intermittent fasting might not be your best option. The truth is that intermittent fasting places stress on the body just like regular exercise does, which increases the cortisol levels produced. By staying well-hydrated throughout the day, you might be able to lessen this effect by making it easier for your body to remove toxins. Although this may appear to be terrible news at first glance, it is only a minor inconvenience, especially for those who want to combine intermittent fasting with regular yoga. As we've shown, yoga reduces our bodies' cortisol, so you can effectively counteract any negative that a non-yoga student could otherwise experience. In conclusion, while intermittent fasting alone cannot be considered useful in reducing stress when paired with yoga, there shouldn't be any negative effects. Besides, things will get much easier when your body adjusts to the new routine and you start to lose weight due to your efforts.

Chapter 3: Breakfast Recipes For Intermittent Fasting

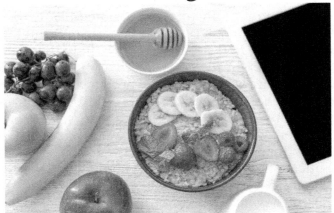

3.1 Warm Roasted Vegetable Farro Salad

Ready in: 1hr 35mins
Serves: 4
Yield: 4
Ingredients
- One tablespoon kosher salt or One tablespoon sea salt
- 1/2 medium-sized eggplant, peel on, and large diced
- One cup cherry tomatoes washed and left whole
- Six white button mushrooms, quartered
- One medium-sized zucchini, peel on and large diced
- Six garlic cloves, peeled, trimmed, and sliced
- 1/2 medium-sized red onion, peeled and cut into wedges
- 1 cup cracked farro
- 2 cups almond milk (Almond Breeze)
- One tablespoon olive oil
- One teaspoon tbsp olive oil (15 mL)
- One tablespoon balsamic vinegar

- 3 sprigs fresh cilantro
- One tablespoon olive oil
- 1/2 teaspoon salt
- 1/2 teaspoon pepper

Instructions

Preheat the oven to 200 C (400 °F). Salt the eggplant slices generously on all sides in a wide flat pan or baking sheet, toss to cover evenly, and keep for 30 minutes to release excess moisture and bitterness. Drain the eggplant and rinse and toss it into a large mixing bowl. Tomatoes, zucchini, mushrooms, garlic, and onions are added. Drizzle the vegetables with olive oil generously, season with salt and pepper, and stir to coat. Move the vegetables to a pan lined with ovenproof tin foil. In the oven, roast the vegetables for 20 - 25 minutes or until tender, caramelized, and forked. To avoid sticking to the plate, stir or flip the vegetables about 10 to 15 minutes into the roasting process. Set aside and remove the pan from the oven. Meanwhile, rinse the farro with water and drain over the sink in a colander. Into a 3-quart (3L) saucepot, add the farro, and add in the Almond Breeze. A pinch of salt and a drizzle of olive oil is added. Bring the liquid to a boil over medium-high heat to prevent boiling, then turn the heat down to a gentle simmer. Simmer the farro with the lid on the pot cocked to one side for 20 minutes to let out steam. Turn off the heat but leave the pot and close the lid on the stovetop. For another 5 minutes or until the farro is soft yet slightly chewy in the middle, steam in the pot. Using a fork to loosen the lid and the fluff. Mix the cooked farro with the vegetables in a large serving dish and gently toss to mix until ready to assemble the dish. Whisk the balsamic vinegar along with the olive oil and drizzle over the farro salad. Toss to coat and season to taste with salt and pepper. Add fresh cilantro and a squeeze of lemon to garnish. Serve it sweet.

3.2 Cajun Potato, Prawn/Shrimp And Avocado Salad
Ready in: 30mins
Serves: 2
Ingredients
- One tablespoon olive oil
- 300 g new potatoes (small baby or chats 10 oz halved)
- 250 g king prawns (8 oz, cooked and peeled)
- Two spring onions (finely sliced)
- One garlic clove (minced)
- Two teaspoons cajun seasoning
- 1 cup alfalfa sprout
- 1 avocado (peeled, stoned, and diced)
- Salt (to boil potatoes)

Instructions

Cook the potatoes for 10 to 15 minutes in a large saucepan of lightly salted boiling water, or until tender, then drain well. In a wok or a large nonstick frying pan/skillet, heat the oil. Season with the prawns, garlic, spring onions, and cajun and fry for 2 to 3 minutes or until the prawns are hot. Stir in the potatoes, then cook for an additional minute. Transfer to dishes for serving and top with the avocado and sprouts of alfalfa and eat.

3.3 Baked Mahi Mahi
Ready in: 40mins
Serves: 4
Ingredients
- 2 lbs mahi-mahi (4 fillets)
- 1/4 teaspoon garlic salt
- One lemon, juiced
- 1 cup mayonnaise
- 1/4 cup white onion, finely chopped
- 1/4 teaspoon ground black pepper
- Breadcrumbs

Instructions

Preheat the oven to 425 degrees. Put it in a baking dish and rinse the fish. Squeeze the fish with lemon juice and sprinkle with garlic, salt, and pepper. Combine the mayonnaise and the chopped onions and scatter them over the fish. Sprinkle with breadcrumbs and bake for 25 minutes at 425°F.

3.4 Sheet Pan Chicken And Brussels Sprouts

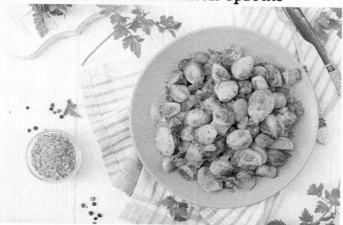

Ready in: 40mins
Serves: 4
Ingredients
- 1 1/2 cups Brussels sprouts, halved
- Four skin-on chicken thighs
- Four carrots, cut on the bias
- One teaspoon herbs de Provence
- Three tablespoons olive oil

Instructions
1. Preheat the stove to 400o F. Put the cut vegetables in a bowl and add 1 1/2 tablespoons of olive oil, 1/2 tablespoons of herbs, salt, and pepper. Rub the vegetables all over.
2. On a sheet pan, place the veggies. In the same bowl, add the chicken thighs. Drizzle with 1 1/2 tablespoons of olive oil, 1/2 tablespoons of herbs, salt, and pepper. Rub the chicken all over.

3. Put the chicken in a pan. Roast for 30-35 minutes or until you're done with the chicken. Turn the oven over to broil and cook for a minute or two if you prefer a crispier vegetable or chicken skin. Carefully watch, or it'll burn.

3.5 Perfect Cauliflower Pizza Crust

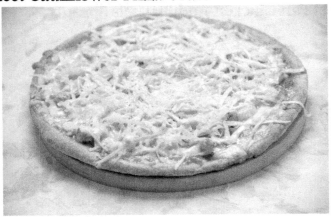

Ready in: 1hr 10mins
Serves: 4

Ingredients

- One egg, beaten
- Four cups raw cauliflower, riced, or one medium cauliflower head
- One cup chevre cheese or 1 cup other soft cheese
- One pinch salt
- One teaspoon dried oregano

Instructions

1. Preheat to 400°F in your oven. Pulse batches of raw cauliflower florets in a food processor to render the cauliflower rice until a rice-like texture are achieved. Fill a big pot and bring it to a boil with around an inch of water. Connect the "rice" and cover; cook for 5 minutes or so. Drain the strainer into a fine-mesh one.

2. **THIS IS THE SECRET:** Move it to a clean, thin dishtowel once you've strained the rice. In the dishtowel, cover the steamed rice, curl it and Suck out all the excess moisture! It's amazing how much extra liquid will be released, leaving you with a good dry crust of the pizza.
3. Mix your strained rice, beaten egg, goat's cheese, and spices in a big bowl. (Don't fear using your hands! You want it mixed well.) It's not going to be like every pizza dough you've ever dealt with, yet don't worry, it's going to stay together!
4. On a baking sheet lined with parchment paper, press the dough out. Keep the dough about 3/8" thick, and make the edges a little higher for a "crust" effect, if you like. Bake at 400 ° for 35-40 minutes.
5. Add sauce, cheese, and any other toppings you want to all your favorites. Put the pizza back in the oven for 400F and bake for an additional 5-10 minutes, only until the cheese is hot and bubbly. Cut and serve!

3.6 Sweet Potato And Black Bean Burrito
Ready in: 1hr 5mins
Yield: 8-12 portions
Ingredients

- 5 cups peeled cubed sweet potatoes
- two teaspoons other vegetable oil or two teaspoons broth
- Half teaspoon salt
- 3 and half cups diced onions
- One tablespoon minced fresh green chili pepper
- 4garlic cloves, minced (or pressed)
- Four teaspoons ground cumin
- 4 and half cups cooked black beans (three 15-ounce cans, drained)
- Four teaspoons ground coriander
- 2/3 cup lightly packed cilantro leaf

- One teaspoon salt
- 12 (10 inches) flour tortillas
- Two tablespoons fresh lemon juice
- Fresh salsa

Instructions

Preheat the oven To 350°. Place the salt and water in a medium saucepan to cover the sweet potatoes. Cover and bring to a boil, then simmer for about 10 minutes, until tender. Drain yourself and set aside. Heat the oil in a medium saucepan or skillet while the sweet potatoes are frying, and add the onions, garlic, and chili. On medium-low heat, cover and cook, occasionally stirring, until the onions are tender, around 7 minutes. Add cumin and coriander and cook, constantly stirring, for 2 to 3 minutes longer. Remove and set aside from the sun. Combine the black beans, lemon juice, cilantro, salt, and cooked sweet potatoes in a food processor and puree until smooth (or mash the ingredients in a large bowl by hand). In a large mixing bowl, pass the sweet potato mixture and blend in the cooked onions and spices. Oil a large baking dish lightly. At the center of each tortilla, spoon around 2/3 to 3/4 cup of the filling, roll it up, and put it in the baking dish, seam side down. Cover thoroughly with foil and bake for 30 minutes or so, until sweet. Serve with salsa topping.

3.7 Sweet Potato Curry With Spinach And Chickpeas

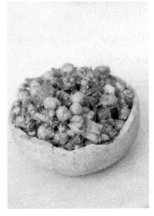

Ready in: 30mins
Serves: 6
Ingredients
- 1 -2 teaspoon canola oil
- One tablespoon cumin
- Two tablespoons curry powder
- One teaspoon cinnamon
- Half large sweet onions, chopped or two scallions, thinly sliced
- Ten ounces fresh spinach washed, stemmed, and coarsely chopped
- One (14 1/2 ounce) can chickpeas, rinsed and drained
- Two large sweet potatoes, peeled and diced (about 2 lbs)
- Half cup water
- 1/4 cup chopped fresh cilantro for garnish
- One (14 1/2 ounce) can diced tomatoes, can substitute fresh if available
- Basmati rice or brown rice, for serving

Instructions
Heat 1-2 tsp of canola or vegetable oil over medium heat while the sweet potatoes are cooking. Add the onions and sauté for 2-3 minutes, or until tender. Add the curry powder, cumin, and cinnamon, then stir to cover the spices' onions evenly. Stir in the tomatoes and their juices, and stir in the chickpeas to blend. Add half a cup of water and lift the heat for about a minute or two to a high simmer. Then add fresh spinach, stirring to cover with cooking liquid, a few handfuls at a time. Cover and boil until just wilted, about 3 minutes, when all the spinach is added to the pan. Apply to the liquid the cooked sweet potatoes, and stir to coat. Simmer for another 3-5 minutes, or until you mix the flavors well. Move to a dish for serving, toss with fresh cilantro and serve sweet. This dish is served beautifully over basmati or brown rice.

3.8 Poached Eggs & Avocado Toasts

Ready in: 15mins
Serves: 4
Ingredients

- Two ripe avocados
- Four eggs
- Two teaspoons lemon juice (or juice of 1 lime)
- One cup cheese (grated, edam, gruyere, or whatever you have on hand)
- Four slices thick bread
- Four teaspoons butter (for spreading on toast)
- Salt & freshly ground black pepper

Instructions

Using your favorite technique, poach eggs. Meanwhile, the avocados are cut in half, and the stones are removed. Scoop out the flesh in a bowl with a spoon and apply the lemon or lime juice and salt & pepper. Mash using a fork. Bread toast and spread with butter. On each slice of buttered toast, spread the avocado mix and top each one with a poached egg. Sprinkle the grated cheese over it and serve immediately. These are also good with tomato halves on the side, either fresh or grilled.

3.9 French Vanilla Almond Granola

Ready in: 2hrs 10mins
Serves: 12
Yield: 12 1/2 cup servings
Ingredients

- Half cup sliced almonds
- 3 and half cups old fashioned oats
- Half cup water
- 1/4 teaspoon salt
- 1/2 cup natural cane sugar
- One tablespoon vanilla extract

- 1/4 cup organic canola oil or 1/4 cup grapeseed oil

Instructions
1. Heat the oven to 200°. Use parchment paper to line a big, rimmed cookie sheet.
2. Combine the oats and the almonds in a dish.
3. Stir the sugar and salt into the water in a small saucepan over medium heat. Stir and cook until the sugar has dissolved. Withdraw from the sun. Stir in the vanilla and canola oil. Pour the oat and almond mixture into the mixture and stir until well mixed. On the lined cookie sheet, spread the mixture out and bake for 2 hours, or until tender to the touch. Oh, don't stir! Remove from the oven and allow to cool into chunks before breaking apart. Store in a bag that is air-tight.

3.10 Vegan Fried 'Fish' Tacos
Ready in: 50mins
Yield: 8 small tacos
Ingredients
- 14 ounces silken tofu
- 1/2 cup plain flour
- 2 cups panko breadcrumbs
- Half teaspoon salt
- Half teaspoon cayenne pepper
- One teaspoon smoked paprika
- One teaspoon ground cumin
- Half cup non-dairy milk
- 1/4 head cabbage, finely shredded
- Vegetable oil, for frying
- One ripe avocado
- Vegan mayonnaise, to serve
- Eight small tortillas

Pickled Onion

- One red onion, peeled, finely sliced
- One tablespoon sugar
- 1/4 cup apple cider vinegar
- One teaspoon salt

Instructions
1. To extract surplus moisture, pat the tofu with a few pieces of kitchen roll. I want them to be imperfect, not cubes, because they look better! Use a knife to split the tofu into rough 1 inch pieces.
2. Place the breadcrumbs in a shallow, large cup. In another large, shallow cup, place the flour, salt, smoked paprika, cayenne, and cumin and stir together.
3. Put the milk in a shallow bowl that is third deep. Take the pieces of tofu and gently coat them on a baking sheet with the flour, then the milk, then the breadcrumbs.
4. Fill a deep frying pan with vegetable oil about 1/2-inch deep. Sprinkle a breadcrumb in, and if it starts to bubble and brown, the oil is hot enough. Put it over medium heat and let the oil get hot. To the oil, add chunks of breaded tofu and fry until golden underneath, then flip and cook so that it's all golden. Remove to a baking sheet lined with a drainable kitchen roll. Repeat with the tofu that remains.

For the pickled onion: Heat the vinegar, salt, and sugar from the apple cider in a small pot until steaming. Put the finely sliced red onion in a bowl or pot and pour the hot vinegar over it. To soften and turn pink, let it sit for at least 30 minutes. Serve the spicy fried tofu, pickled onion, a smear of vegan mayo, some avocado, and shredded cabbage in warmed tortillas (I warm them over my stove's lit gas ring).

Chapter 4: Lunch Recipes For Intermittent Fasting

4.1 Mama's Supper Club Tilapia Parmesan

Ready in: 35mins
Serves: 4

Ingredients

- Half cup grated parmesan cheese
- Two tablespoons lemon juice
- Three tablespoons mayonnaise
- Three tablespoons finely chopped green onions
- Four tablespoons butter, room temperature
- 1/4 teaspoon dried basil
- black pepper
- 1/4 teaspoon seasoning salt (I like Old Bay seasoning here)
- One dash of hot pepper sauce
- 2 lbs tilapia fillets (orange roughy, cod, or red snapper can be substituted)

Instructions

Preheat the oven to 350°C. Lay the fillets in a single layer in a buttered 13-by-9-inch baking dish or jelly roll pan. Do not have fillets stacked. Brush with juice on top. Mix the cheese, butter, mayonnaise, onions, and seasonings in a dish. Blend well with the fork. In a preheated oven, bake the fish for 10 to 20 minutes or until the fish just begins to flake. Spread with cheese mixture and bake for around 5 minutes, until golden brown. Baking time will depend on the fish thickness that you are using. Control the fish carefully so that they do not overcook.

Note: You can make this fish in a broiler, too.
Broil for 3-4 minutes or until nearly through.
Attach the cheese and broil for 2 to 3 minutes or until it is browned.

4.2 Shredded Brussels Sprouts With Bacon And Onions

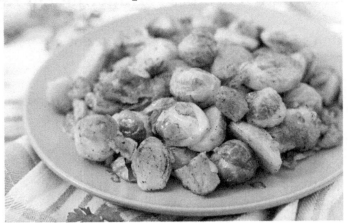

Ready in: 30mins
Serves: 6
Ingredients
- One small yellow onion, thinly sliced
- Two slices of bacon
- 3/4 cup water
- One teaspoon Dijon mustard
- 1/4 teaspoon salt (or to taste)
- One tablespoon cider vinegar
- 1 lb Brussels sprout, trimmed, halved, and very thinly sliced

Instructions
Cook bacon in a pan until crisp (5 to 7 minutes) over medium heat; drain on paper towels, then crumble. Transfer the onion and salt to the pan's drippings and cook over medium heat until tender and browned, frequently stirring (about 3 minutes). Add water and mustard, scrape any browned parts, add sprouts from Brussels and cook, stirring regularly, until tender (4 to 6 minutes). Stir in the vinegar and add the crumbled bacon to the tip.

4.3 Roasted Broccoli With Lemon Garlic & Toasted Pine Nuts

Ready in: 22mins
Serves: 4

Ingredients

- 1 lb broccoli floret
- salt & freshly ground black pepper
- Two tablespoons olive oil
- Two tablespoons unsalted butter
- Half teaspoon lemon zest, grated
- One teaspoon garlic, minced
- 1 ~2 tablespoon fresh lemon juice
- Two tablespoons pine nuts, toasted

Instructions

Preheat the oven to 500°C. Toss the broccoli with the oil in a wide bowl and add salt and pepper to taste. On a baking sheet, arrange the florets into a single layer and roast, turning once for 12 minutes or until just tender. Meanwhile, over medium heat, melt the butter in a small saucepan. Apply the zest of garlic and lemon and heat for about 1 minute, stirring. Let the lemon juice cool slightly and stir it in. Put the broccoli in a serving bowl, pour the lemon butter over it, and toss to coat it. Over the top, scatter the toasted pinenuts.

4.4 Cauliflower Popcorn - Roasted Cauliflower

Ready in: 1hr 10mins
Serves: 4

Ingredients

- Four tablespoons olive oil
- One head cauliflower
- One teaspoon salt, to taste

Instructions

Preheat the oven to 425°C.

Trim the cauliflower head, discarding the thick stems and the core; cut the florets into pieces around the ping-pong balls' size. Combine the olive oil and salt in a large bowl, whisk, then add the pieces of cauliflower and toss thoroughly. For quick cleaning, line a baking sheet with parchment (you can skip that, if you don't have one, then spread the cauliflower pieces on the sheet and roast for 1 hour, turning three or four times, until most of each piece turns golden brown (the browner the pieces of cauliflower turn, the more caramelization happens and the sweeter they taste).

4.5 Best Baked Potato
Ready in: 1hr 10mins
Serves: 1
Ingredients
- Canola oil
- One large russet potato
- Kosher salt

Instructions
Heat the oven to 350 ° F and place the upper and lower thirds of the racks. Thoroughly wash the potato (or potatoes) with a stiff brush and cold running water. Dry, then poke 8 to 12 deep holes all over the spud using a regular fork so that moisture can escape during cooking. Place it in a bowl and gently coat it with oil. Sprinkle with kosher salt and put the potato in the middle of the oven directly on a rack. To trap any drippings, place a baking sheet (I placed a piece of aluminum foil) on the lower rack. Bake for 1 hour or until the skin feels crisp, but the flesh feels soft underneath. Serve by forming a dotted line with your fork from end to end, then crack the spud open by pressing the ends towards each other. It's going to pop open right. But watch out, there's going to be some steam there. **Note:** You will need to increase the cooking time by up to 15 minutes if you are cooking more than four potatoes.

4.6 Easy Black Bean Soup

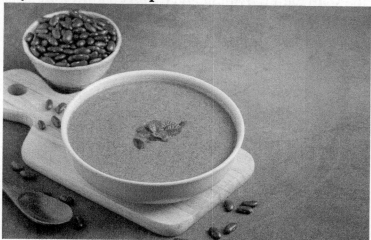

Ready in: 25mins
Serves: 4

Ingredients

- Three tablespoons olive oil
- One tablespoon ground cumin
- One medium onion, chopped
- 2 ~3 cloves garlic
- Two (14 1/2 ounce) cans of black beans
- Salt and pepper
- Two cups chicken broth or 2 cups vegetable broth
- One small red onion, chopped fine
- 1/4 cup cilantro, coarsely chopped or finely chopped (whatever you prefer)

Instructions

In olive oil, saute the onion. Add cumin when the onion becomes translucent. Cook for 30 seconds, add garlic, and cook for an additional 30 to 60 seconds. Add one can of vegetable broth and 2 cups of black beans. Bring to a boil, sometimes stirring. Turn the heat off. Mix the ingredients in the pot using a hand blender, or switch them to a blender. Connect the second can of beans and the mixed ingredients to the pot and bring to a simmer. Serve the soup with red onion bowls and cilantro for garnishing.

4.7 Vegan Lentil Burger

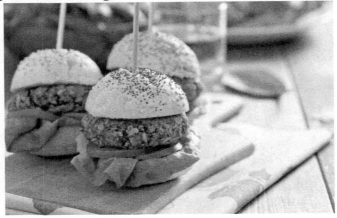

Ready in: 1hr 10mins
Yield: 8-10 burgers

Ingredients
- 2 and half cups water
- 1 cup dry lentils, well rinsed
- Half teaspoon salt
- Half medium onion, diced
- One carrot, diced
- One tablespoon olive oil
- One teaspoon pepper
- One tablespoon soy sauce
- 3/4 cup breadcrumbs
- 3/4 cup rolled oats, finely ground

Instructions
Boil the lentils with the salt in the water for about 45 minutes. The lentils are going to be soft, and much of the water is gone. It will take about 5 minutes to fry the onions and carrots in oil

until tender. The cooked ingredients are combined in a bowl with pepper, soy sauce, oats, and bread crumbs. While the mixture is still warm, it will produce ten burgers. Burgers can then be fried shallowly on each side for 1-2 minutes or baked for 15 minutes at 200C.

4.8 Vegan Coconut Kefir Banana Muffins

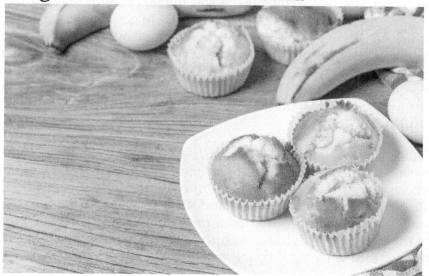

Ready in: 45mins
Serves: 12
Ingredients

- 2 cups all-purpose flour
- One cup unsweetened dried shredded coconut
- One cup granulated sugar
- Two teaspoons baking soda
- Half teaspoon salt
- Two ripe bananas, mashed
- One teaspoon baking powder
- 1/4 cup cold-pressed liquid coconut oil

- 1 and half cups pc dairy-free kefir probiotic fermented coconut milk
- One teaspoon vanilla extract

Instructions

Preheat the oven to 180oC (350oF).

Mist 12-Count Cooking Spray Muffin Tin. Only set aside. In a big bowl, whisk together the flour, sugar, coconut, baking soda, baking powder, and salt. Only set aside. In a separate, large cup, whisk together the bananas, kefir, coconut oil, and vanilla. Add to the flour mixture; stir until there are no white streaks left. Divide the prepared muffin tin between the wells. Cook until the tops are golden and the toothpick inserted in the centers comes out clean, about 30 minutes. Let it cool for 15 minutes in the muffin pan.

Chef's tip: let them cool fully on a rack to freeze muffins, then move to an airtight container or resealable freezer bag and freeze for up to a month. You may individually cover the muffins in plastic wrap or foil before placing them in the container or bag for additional protection against freezer burn. In the oven, Overnight thaw muffins or microwave straight from frozen until warmed through around 20 to 30 seconds.

4.9 Sauerkraut Salad

Ready in: 15mins
Serves: 6

Ingredients

- 1 cup celery, chopped fine
- 1 (1 lb) can sauerkraut, drained but not rinsed
- Half cup green pepper, chopped fine
- Half teaspoon salt
- Two tablespoons onions, chopped fine
- Half teaspoon pepper
- 1/3 cup salad oil
- 3/4 cup sugar

- 1/3 cup cider (I use white) or 1/3 cup white vinegar (I use white)

Instructions

Mix the sauerkraut with the chopped vegetables. On low heat, heat the sugar, oil, vinegar, salt, and pepper until the sugar dissolves. Refrigerate and pour over the vegetables. Overnight relax.

4.10 Spicy Chocolate Keto Fat Bombs

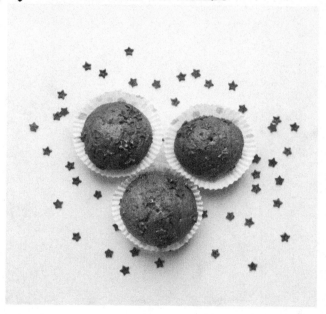

Ready in: 8mins
Serves: 24

Ingredients

- 2/3 cup coconut oil
- Half cup dark cocoa
- 4 (6 g) packets stevia (or to taste)
- 2/3 cup smooth peanut butter
- One tablespoon ground cinnamon
- Half cup toasted coconut flakes

- 1/4 teaspoon kosher salt
- 1/4 teaspoon cayenne (to taste)

Instructions

In a double boiler set over a pot of simmering water, blend the coconut oil, peanut butter, and cocoa powder. Heat, whisking, until smooth and molten. To mix, add stevia, cinnamon, and salt and stir. Divide the mixture into a mini muffin tray made of silicone. Top with coconut and cayenne and move to the freezer for about 30 minutes, until solid.

Chapter 5: Dinner Recipes For Intermittent Fasting

5.1 Zucchini And Eggs Recipe With Cheese
Cook Time: 16 min
Prep Time: 4 min
Total Time: 20 min
Servings: 1
Ingredients
- One yellow onion small, sliced thinly, about 4 ounces
- One tablespoon olive oil separated
- 2-3 garlic cloves sliced in half
- One small zucchini chopped into ½-inch quarters (see note), about 6 ounces
- One egg room temperature, slightly beaten
- Salt and pepper to taste
- One tablespoon water
- One tablespoon Italian parsley chopped
- 1-2 tablespoons Romano cheese grated

Instructions
1. Heat 1/2 tablespoons of olive oil over medium-high heat in a large skillet. Add the onion and reduce to medium heat.
2. Cook, stirring until translucent periodically and softened for around 3-5 minutes.
3. The remaining chopped zucchini, olive oil, and garlic are added. With salt and pepper, season.
4. Saute, stirring and shaking the pan, until golden brown, over medium-high heat. It should take about 7-10 minutes for this. The zucchini needs to be baked, but it's still crisp—taste of doneness. If necessary, change the heat.
5. Meanwhile, whisk the cheese and parsley with the egg.
6. Add the egg mixture to the pan when the zucchini is cooked, and let it cook for about 30 seconds. Then stir and shake the pan until the egg is scrambled and set for 1 minute or so.
7. Taste the seasonings and change. Immediately serve. Garnish with chopped Italian parsley and grated cheese, if needed.

Nutrition: 1serving | Carbohydrates: 17g | Calories: 280kcal | Protein: 10g | Fat: 20g | Saturated Fat: 4g | Sodium: 141mg | Potassium: 529mg | Cholesterol: 169mg | Fiber: 3g | Sugar: 8g | Iron: 2mg Vitamin A: 811IU | Vitamin C: 36mg | Calcium: 133mg

5.2 Egg Scramble With Sweet Potatoes
Ingredients:

- ½ cup chopped onion
- One (8-oz) sweet potato, diced
- 2 tsp chopped rosemary
- Salt
- Four large eggs
- Four large egg whites
- Pepper
- 2 tbsp chopped chive

Instructions
Preheat the heater to 425 degrees F. Toss the sweet potato, onion, rosemary, salt, and pepper on a baking dish. Spray with cooking spray and roast for about 20 minutes, until tender. Meanwhile, whisk the eggs, egg whites, and a pinch of salt and pepper together in a medium cup. Spritz a cooking spray skillet and scramble the eggs over medium heat for around 5 minutes. Sprinkle and serve with the spuds with chopped chives.
Nutrition: 571 calories per serving, 44 g of protein, 52 g of carbohydrates (9 g of fibre), 20 g of fat

5.3 Spicy Spanish Tomato Baked Eggs
Ingredients

- One tbsp olive oil
- One red pepper, deseeded and cut into strips
- Two red onions, peeled and cut into half-moons
- One clove garlic, peeled and sliced
- 1 tsp paprika

- Four medium eggs
- 250g cherry tomatoes, halved or one tin peeled plum tomatoes
- Two tbsp chopped flat-leaf parsley (optional)

Instructions

1. Preheat the oven to 180 ° C. Heat the oil in a large, deep, ovenproof frying pan. Add the onions, garlic, and pepper. Season with freshly ground black pepper and cook until soft or for 10 minutes. Add the tomatoes and paprika and cook gently for an additional 5 minutes.
2. In the mixture, make four little wells and crack an egg into each. Season, cover, and place in the oven with black pepper.
3. Cook until the eggs are set - this should take 5-8 minutes or so. If used, sprinkle over the parsley.

5.4 Vegetable Meatloaf With Balsamic Glaze

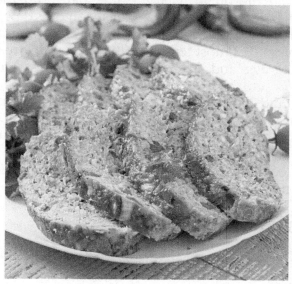

Ingredients
- Two tablespoons extra-virgin olive oil
- One small zucchini, finely diced

- One large egg, lightly beaten
- One red bell pepper, finely diced
- One yellow bell pepper, finely diced
- Five cloves garlic smashed to a paste with coarse salt
- Kosher salt and freshly ground pepper
- 1/4 cup chopped fresh parsley
- 1/2 cup Parmesan cheese or freshly grated Romano
- 1 1/2 pounds ground turkey (90% lean)
- 1 cup panko (coarse Japanese breadcrumbs)
- One tablespoon finely chopped fresh thyme
- 1/4 cup plus two tablespoons balsamic vinegar
- 3/4 cup ketchup

Instructions

The oven should be preheated to 425 degrees. Over high pressure, heat the oil in a large saute pan. Add the zucchini, garlic paste, bell peppers, and 1/4 teaspoon of red pepper flakes. Season with pepper and salt and cook for about 5 minutes, until the vegetables are almost tender. Set to cool aside. In a large cup, whisk in the egg and fresh herbs. Add turkey, panko, grated cheese, 1/2 cup of ketchup, two tablespoons of cooled vegetables, and balsamic vinegar; blend until just mixed. Press the mixture into a 9-by-5-inch loaf pan gently. In a small bowl, whisk the remaining 1/4 cup balsamic vinegar and1/4 cup ketchup, 1/4 teaspoon red pepper flakes; brush the blend over the whole loaf. For 1 to 1 1/4 hours, bake. Until slicing, let it rest for 10 minutes.

5.5 Easy Bbq Chicken Tostadas

Prep Time: 10 min
Total Time: 18 min
Cook Time: 8 min
Servings: 4

Ingredients

- Three cups cooked and shredded chicken
- One and half cups of your favorite barbecue sauce, divided

- Eight tostada shells or eight corn tortillas brushed lightly with olive oil and baked for 3-5 minutes per side, until crispy
- Three green onions, very thinly sliced (optional)
- Two cups shredded cheese (Mary uses mozzarella in the cookbook, but I have also used cheddar, Monterey Jack, or a blend)

Instructions

Preheat to 350°F in your oven. Spread out two rimmed baking sheets with the tostada shells (or baked tortillas). In a small bowl, mix the chicken and 1 cup barbecue sauce, and swirl to coat. Divide the chicken between the shells of the tostada and top with the cheese (approximately 1/4 cup each). Bake, only until the cheese is melted, for 6 to 8 minutes. Remove and drizzle with the remaining 1/2 cup of barbecue sauce from the oven. If needed, sprinkle it with green onions.

5.6 Buffalo Chicken Sandwich With Blue Cheese Slaw
Ingredients
Blue Cheese Slaw:
- 1/4 cup mayonnaise
- One tablespoon minced garlic
- 1/4 cup crumbled blue cheese
- Two tablespoons Worcestershire sauce
- 1 (10-ounce) package coleslaw mix
- Kosher salt
- One lemon, juiced
- Freshly cracked black pepper
- Canola oil, to fry

Buffalo Chicken:
- Half cup buffalo hot sauce, store-bought
- Two tablespoons smoked paprika, plus more for seasoning
- 4 (6-ounce) boneless, skinless chicken cutlets
- One tablespoon kosher salt, plus more for seasoning

- One cup self-rising flour
- One and 1/4 cups buttermilk
- Two tablespoons hot sauce
- One egg
- One tablespoon cracked black pepper, plus more for seasoning
- Four soft-club rolls, split and toasted

Instructions

1. Mix the mayonnaise, crumbled blue cheese, garlic, Worcestershire sauce, and lemon juice in a medium-sized bowl until well mixed. Attach the mix of coleslaw and toss well. With salt and pepper, season and set aside.
2. Heat enough canola oil in a deep-fryer or heavy-bottomed pot to get halfway up the sides of the pot to 350 degrees F.
3. In a shallow dish, add buffalo sauce and set aside. To taste, season the chicken with smoked paprika and salt and pepper. In a shallow dish, place the flour, two tablespoons of paprika, one tablespoon of salt, and one tablespoon of pepper. Put the egg, buttermilk, and hot sauce together in another shallow dish and whisk together. Dredge each piece of chicken, shake off any excess in the buttermilk mixture, and then dredge it into the flour mixture. Fry until the chicken is cooked for around 4 to 6 minutes. On an instant-read thermometer, the internal temperature registers 165 degrees F. In the buffalo sauce, dip the finished chicken and place it on the club rolls. Top the chicken and shape a sandwich with a liberal quantity of slaw.

5.7 Italian Chicken

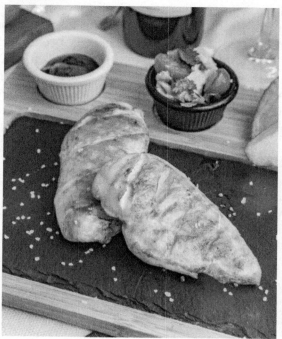

Cook Time: 30 min
Prep Time: 10 min
Ingredients

- Four boneless skinless chicken breasts
- Half cup breadcrumbs
- Half cup grated parmesan cheese
- Half teaspoon minced garlic
- Salt and pepper to taste
- Four tablespoons butter melted
- One teaspoon Italian seasoning
- 1 pound small potatoes halved or quartered
- Cooking spray
- Two tablespoons chopped parsley

- Lemon wedges optional garnish

Instructions

To 400 degrees, preheat the oven. Using cooking spray to cover a sheet pan. Mix the parmesan cheese, breadcrumbs, garlic, Italian seasoning, salt, and pepper in a small cup. In the melted butter, dip the top of each chicken breast, then press the chicken's top into the breadcrumb mixture to coat it. On the prepared sheet pan, put the chicken breasts. About the chicken, scatter the potatoes. Drizzle over the potatoes and chicken with the remaining butter. With salt and pepper, season the potatoes. Bake for 25-30 minutes or until the chicken is completely cooked and the potatoes are tender. Depending on the thickness of your chicken, the cooking time can vary. Sprinkle and serve with parsley. If needed, garnish with lemon wedges.

5.8 Oriental Turkey Burger

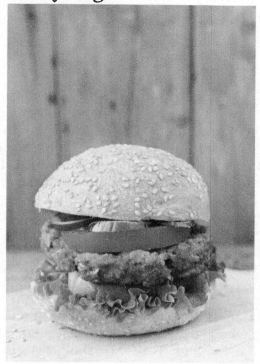

Ingredients
SLAW:

- 2 cups coleslaw mix
- One tablespoon seasoned rice vinegar
- Three tablespoons chopped fresh cilantro
- One teaspoon vegetable oil

BURGER:

- Two tablespoons Butter
- Two jalapeño chile peppers, seeded, finely chopped
- 1/3 cup chopped green onions
- 1 1/4 pounds lean ground turkey
- One tablespoon hoisin sauce

- One tablespoon soy sauce
- 1/4 cup dry bread crumbs
- One tablespoon butter, melted
- Hoisin sauce, if desired
- 5 (10-inch) tortillas

Instructions

Heat the gas grill until the coals are ash white on a medium or charcoal grill. In a tub, mix all the slaw ingredients; mix well. Cover; leave to cool before serving time. Melt two tablespoons of butter until sizzling in a 10-inch skillet; add the onion and chili peppers. Cook for approximately 1-2 minutes or until tender. Cool. In a cup, combine the onion mix, turkey, bread crumbs, one tablespoon of hoisin sauce, and soy sauce; mix gently. Shape into four patties (3/4 inches thick). Set the patties on the grill— a molten butter brush. Grill, rotating once, 20-30 minutes or until the inner temperature reaches a minimum of 165 °f and the middle of the meat is no longer pink. Wrap the aluminum foil tortillas. Place them away from direct heat on the grill. Move tortillas often when grilling burgers. Place half of each warm tortilla with the burgers. Top with slaw; drizzle, if necessary, with hoisin sauce. Fold your tortilla over your burger.

5.9 Easy Shepherd's Pie Recipe

Cook time: 50 minutes
Prep time: 15 minutes

Ingredients

- 8 Tablespoons (1 stick) butter
- 1 1/2 to 2 pounds potatoes (about three large potatoes), peeled and quartered
- One medium onion, chopped (about 1 1/2 cups)
- 1 1/2 lbs ground round beef
- 1-2 cups vegetables—diced carrots, corn, peas
- Half cup beef broth
- Salt, pepper, other seasonings of choice

- One teaspoon Worcestershire sauce

Instructions

Boil the potatoes: Place the peeled and quartered potatoes in a medium-sized bath. Cover for at least an inch with cold water. There is a teaspoon of salt added. Bring to a boil, simmer, and cook, then reduce to a simmer until tender (about 20 minutes). Sauté vegetables: Melt four tablespoons of butter over medium heat in a large saucepan while frying the potatoes. Attach the chopped onions and cook them until tender for approximately 6 to 10 minutes. Add them if you have vegetables, according to their cooking time. Carrots should be baked with onions, as they take as long to cook as onions.

Add them at the end of the onion cooking process or after the meat starts to cook if peas or corn are included, as they take very little time to cook. Add the ground beef and then the Worcestershire sauce and the broth: add the onions and vegetables to the ground beef pan. Cook until there's no pinker. With salt and pepper, season. Add the beef broth and Worcestershire sauce. Simmer the broth and reduce the heat to a low level. To prevent the meat from drying out, cook uncovered for 10 minutes, adding more beef broth if necessary. Mash the cooked potatoes: When the potatoes are cooked, remove them from the pot and put them in a bowl with the remaining four Teaspoons of butter (a fork will easily pierce). With a fork or potato masher, mash and season to taste with salt and pepper. Arrange the meat mixture in a casserole dish with the mashed potatoes: Preheat the oven to 400 °F. In a bread baking dish, spread the beef, onions, and vegetables (if used) in an even layer (9×1 casserole). On top of the ground beef, spread the mashed potatoes over the top. Using a fork to rough up the mashed potatoes' surface so that there are peaks that get well browned. You can also use a fork to render the mashed potatoes with innovative designs. Bake in the oven: Put in the oven at 400°F and cook for about 30 minutes until browned and bubbling.

5.10 Spaghetti Diablo with Shrimp

Prep Time: 5 minutes   **Cook Time:** 25 minutes   **Servings:** 4

Ingredients

- ½ teaspoon olive oil

- Half onion, chopped

- One can of diced tomatoes

- ¼ cup white wine

- 6 ounces cooked shrimp

- Salt and ground black pepper

- Half green bell pepper, chopped

- ¼ cup grated Pecorino-Romano cheese

- Half yellow bell pepper, chopped

- 4 ounces' spaghetti

- ¼ teaspoon dried oregano

- 3 cloves garlic, crushed

- ¼ teaspoon red pepper flakes

- ¼ cup chopped fresh parsley, divided

- ¼ teaspoon dried basil

Instructions

In a Dutch oven, heat the oil over medium-high heat. 5 to 7 minutes in heated oil, stir and cook yellow bell pepper, green bell pepper, onions, and garlic until soft. Season with salt & pepper. Bring the bell pepper combination to a boil with the tomatoes, alcohol, 1/4 cup parsley, oregano, basil and red pepper flakes; lower heat to low and cover the Dutch oven.

Cook, stirring regularly, for approximately 2 hours, or until the tomatoes have broken down. Bring a big saucepan of water to a boil, lightly salted. Cook spaghetti in boiling water for approximately 10 minutes. Cook, occasionally stirring, until the drained pasta and shrimp are fully cooked but still stiff to the touch, 2 to 4 minutes longer. Toss with the remaining Pecorino-Romano cheese and parsley before serving.

Nutrition: Fat 3.5g; Protein 29g; Sodium 233mg

Chapter 6: Dessert Recipes For Intermittent Fasting

6.1 Citrus Dark Chocolate Mousse

Prep Time: 5 minutes   **Cook Time:** 15 minutes   **Servings:** 5

Ingredients

- One tsp of brewed coffee

- 85g of dark chocolate

- One pinch of rock salt

- One tsp of orange zest

- Half tsp of lime zest

- 3 medium eggs

Instructions

In a small dish, combine orange and lime zest. On top of the double boiler, combine the chocolate and coffee with the zest over warm water. To keep the mixture from bubbling, stir it. Remove the chocolate from the heat after it has melted and set it aside to cool. The egg whites and salt should be whisked together. Stir the egg yolks in the chocolate mixture, then pour the mixture over egg whites and gently fold them in. Make small bowls or glasses out of the mixture. Refrigerate for at least 4 hours before serving.

Nutrition: Fat 36g; Protein 10g; Sodium 294mg;

6.2 Peanut Butter Cookies

Prep Time: 15 minutes
Cook Time: 10 minutes
Servings: 24

Ingredients

- Half teaspoon salt

- 2 large eggs

- 1 ½ teaspoons baking soda

- One cup crunchy peanut butter

- One cup unsalted butter

- One teaspoon baking powder

- One cup white sugar

- 2 ½ cups all-purpose flour

- One cup packed brown sugar

Instructions

In a mixing bowl, combine together cream butter, peanut butter, and sugar; add in the eggs. Mix flour, baking powder, baking soda, and salt in a separate dish, then add the butter mixture. Refrigerate the dough for 1 hour. Make 1 inch balls out of the dough and place them on baking pans. Using a fork, flatten each ball into a crisscross pattern. Bake for approximately 10 minutes in a preheated 375°F oven until the cookies appear brown.

Nutrition: Fat 136g; Protein 4.5g; Sodium 209.4mg

6.3 Mango and Passionfruit Roulade
Prep Time: 20 minutes
Cook Time: 15 minutes
Servings: 4

Ingredients

- 85g of sugar

- 3 eggs

- 250g of frozen raspberries

- 1 tsp of vanilla extract

- One tub of Greek yogurt

- 2 mangoes

- 85g plain flour, sifted

- One tsp baking powder

- One tbsp of sugar

- 2 ripe passion fruits

Instructions

Preheat the oven to 180°C. In a large mixing bowl, mix the eggs and sugar until it's thick and light. After that, fold in the flour and baking powder, followed by the vanilla. Place the mixture in the pan, tilting it to level it out, and bake for 14-15 minutes until it's brown. Place on a new piece of paper that has been powdered with 1 tbsp caster sugar. Allow cooling fully after rolling the paper within the sponge. Fold the sugar, passion fruit pulp, and one-third of the mango and raspberries. Unroll the sponge, spread with filling, then roll-up.

Nutrition: Fat 3g; Protein 5g; Sodium 256mg;

6.4 Strawberry-Chocolate Greek Yogurt

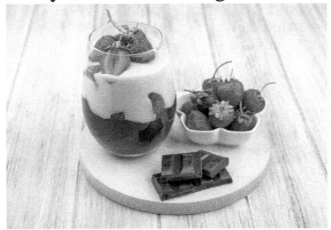

Prep Time: 10 minutes
Cook Time: 180 minutes
Servings: 32
Ingredients

- One cup of sliced strawberries

- 2 tbsp. of honey

- ¼ cup of chocolate chips

- 3 cups plain Greek yogurt

- One teaspoon vanilla extract

Instructions

Using parchment paper, line in a baking sheet. Combine the yogurt, honey, and vanilla extract in a medium mixing bowl. Make a rectangle on the lined baking sheet. Sprinkle the chocolate chips on top and spread the strawberries on top. Freeze for at least 3 hours, or until extremely firm. Cut to pieces to serve.

Nutrition: Fat 1.3g; Protein 2g; Sodium 7.6mg

6.5 Almond Butter Chocolate Chip Cookies
Prep Time: 15 minutes
Cook Time: 35 minutes
Servings: 15
Ingredients

- ¼ cup chopped peanuts

- One egg

- One cup of almond butter

- Half cup of chocolate chips

- One teaspoon of baking soda

- Half cup of brown sugar

Instructions

Preheat the oven to 350°F. Line two baking pans with parchment paper. In a medium mixing bowl, whisk together the egg. Combine almond butter, brown sugar, and baking soda in a mixing bowl and whisk until smooth. Combine peanuts and chocolate chips in a mixing bowl. To create each cookie, take roughly 1 tablespoon of dough and roll it into a compact ball. Place the cookies 1 inch apart on the prepared pan pans. With the tip of a spoon, gently push down on each ball. Bake the cookies for 9 to 10 minutes, or until the tops are cracked, and the edges are brown. Allow cooling for 10 minutes on the pan.

Nutrition: Fat 10g; Protein 4g; Sodium 108mg

Chapter 7: 16/8 INTERMITTENT FASTING PLAN FOR 21 DAYS

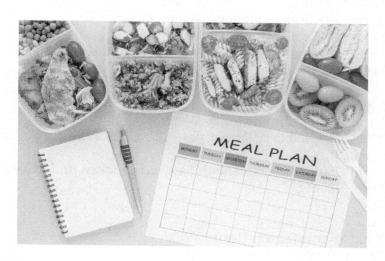

WEEK 1
DAY 1
8: 00am: Warm Lemon Honey Water
11:00 am: Cajun Potato, Prawn/Shrimp And Avocado Salad
3:00 pm: Kind Bar
5:00 pm: Oriental Turkey Burgers, Brown Rice
7:00 pm: Fasting

DAY 2
8:00 am: Warm Lemon Honey Water
11:00 am: Baked Mahi Mahi
3:00 pm: Apple Slices
5:00 pm: Zucchini And Eggs Recipe With Cheese
7:00 pm: Fasting

DAY 3
8:00 am: Warm Lemon Honey Water
11:00 am: Almond Butter/Oatmeal, Coffee/Coconut Creamer
3:00 pm: Nuts
5:00 pm: Tomatoes/Sauteed Egg, Brown Rice

7:00 pm: Fasting

DAY 4
8:00 am: Warm Lemon Honey Water
11:00 am: Coconut Creamer/Coffee, Avocado Toast/Egg
3:00 pm: Banana/Strawberry Smoothie
5:00 pm: Steamed Broccoli, Teriyaki Chicken, Brown Rice
7:00 pm: Fasting

DAY 5
8:00 am: Warm Lemon Honey Water
11:00 am: Triple Berry Smoothies, Coconut Creamer/Coffee
3:00 pm: Nuts
5:00 pm: Cauliflower Rice with Sauteed Chicken and Mushroom
7:00 pm: Fasting

DAY 6
8:00 am: Warm Lemon Honey Water
11:00 am: Whole Wheat Pancake
Coconut Creamer/Coffee
3:00 pm: Blueberries
5:00 pm: Dine Out
7:00 pm: Fasting

DAY 7
8:00 am: Warm Lemon Honey Water
9:00 am: Coconut Milk with Coffee
11:00 am: Skip Breakfast
3:00 pm: Nuts
5:00 pm: Spicy Spanish Tomato Baked Eggs
7:00 pm: Fasting

WEEK 2
DAY 8
8:00 am: Lemon water
8:30 am: Skip breakfast
12:00 pm: Avocado chicken salad
3:00 pm: Nuts
7:00 pm: Easy Bbq Chicken Tostadas
8:00 pm: Begin fasting

DAY 9
8:00 am: Black coffee
8:30 am: Skip breakfast
12:00 pm: Vegan chickpea salad
3:00 pm: Fruit of your choice
7:00 pm: Italian Chicken
8:00 pm: Begin fasting

DAY 10
8:00 am: Black coffee
8:30 am: Skip breakfast
12:00 pm: Tuna avocado salad wrap
3:00 pm: Shredded Brussels Sprouts With Bacon And Onions
7:00 pm: Easy Shepherd's Pie
8:00 pm: Begin fasting

DAY 11
8:00 am: Apple cider vinegar drink
8:30 am: Skip breakfast
12:00 pm: Broccoli tofu salad
3:00 pm: Dark chocolate
7:00 pm: Salmon kale salad
8:00 pm: Begin fasting

DAY 12
8:00 am: Lemon water
8:30 am: Skip breakfast
12:00 pm: Turkey chili
3:00 pm: Roasted Broccoli With Lemon Garlic & Toasted Pine Nuts

7:00 pm: Grilled chicken salad
8:00 pm: Begin fasting

DAY 13
8:00 am: Lemon water
8:30 am: Skip breakfast
12:00 pm: Grilled salmon
3:00 pm: Dark chocolate bark
7:00 pm: Chicken tortilla soup
8:00 pm: Begin fasting

DAY 14
8: 00 am: Black coffee
8:30 am: Skip breakfast
12:00 pm: Vegan Lentil Burgers
3:00 pm: Greek yogurt
7:00 pm: Buffalo Chicken Sandwich With Blue Cheese Slaw
8:00 pm: Begin fasting

WEEK 3
DAY 15
8:00 am: Lemon water
8:30 am: Skip breakfast
12:00 pm: Sauerkraut Salad
3:00 pm: Dark chocolate bark
7:00 pm: Chicken tortilla soup
8:00 pm: Begin fasting

DAY 16
8:00 am: Black coffee
8:30 am: Skip breakfast
12:00 pm: Best Baked Potato
3:00 pm: Handful of nuts
7:00 pm: Easy Bbq Chicken Tostadas
8:00 pm: Begin fasting

Day 17
8:00 am: Lemon water

8:30 am: Skip breakfast
12:00 pm: Chocolate peanut butter shake
3:00 pm: Mama's Supper Club Tilapia Parmesan
7:00 pm: Egg Scramble With Sweet Potatoes
8:00 pm: Begin fasting

Day 18
8:00 am: Apple cider vinegar drink
8:30 am: Skip breakfast
12:00 pm: Tuna Avocado salad wrap
3:00 pm: Roasted Broccoli With Lemon Garlic & Toasted Pine Nuts
7:00 pm: Zucchini And Eggs Recipe With Cheese
8:00 pm: Begin fasting

Day 19
8:00 am: Lemon water
8:30 am: Skip breakfast
12:00 pm: Egg salad
3:00 pm: Piece of dark chocolate
7:00pm: Salmon kale salad
8:00 pm: Begin fasting

Day 20
8:00 am: Black coffee
8:30 am: Skip breakfast
12:00 pm: Turkey chili
3:00 pm: Organic Edamame
7:00 pm: Grilled chicken salad
8:00 pm: Begin fasting

Day 21
8:00 am: Apple cider vinegar drink
12:00 pm: Grilled salmon salad
3:00 pm: Dark chocolate bark
7:00 pm: Vegetable Meatloaf With Balsamic Glaze
8:00 pm: Begin fasting

Conclusion

IF diets have shown some promise in the field of nutrition and health. Additional study is required before we can say with certainty whether the eating pattern is safe over the long run and whether users are likely to stick with it to continue to benefit.

Also, remember that just incorporating fasting days or hours into your eating schedule won't guarantee a healthy diet. Choosing healthy foods on your feasting days is likely to be beneficial to your health. However, if you overindulge on your feast days or eat unhealthier meals, you won't likely experience the positive effects on your health that you wish for.

Made in the USA
Las Vegas, NV
17 May 2023

72179362R00056